Abraham Morgentaler, M.D.

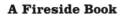

A Fireside Book

Published by Simon & Schuster

New York London Toronto Sydney Tokyo Singapore

THE MALE BODY

a physician's guide to what every man should know about his sexual health

FIRESIDE
Simon & Schuster Building
Rockefeller Center
1230 Avenue of the Americas
New York, New York 10020

FIRESIDE and colophon are registered trademarks
of Simon & Schuster Inc.

Designed by Hyun Joo Kim
Line drawings by Harriet Greenfield
Manufactured in the United States of America

10 9 8 7 6 5 4 3 2 1

Library of Congress Cataloging-in-Publication Data

Morgentaler, Abraham.
    The male body: a physician's guide to what every man
should know about his sexual health/Abraham Morgentaler.
        p.   cm.
    "A Fireside book."
    Includes index.
    1. Andrology—Popular works.   2. Generative organs, Male—
Popular works.   3. Generative organs, Male—Diseases—Case
studies.   I. Title.
RC682.9.M67   1993
612.6'1—dc20   93-18035
                                                              CIP

ISBN 0-671-86426-2

■

This book is dedicated to my mother, Chawa Rosenfarb, who always encouraged the writer in me; and to my father, Henry Morgentaler, M.D., for giving me an appreciation for the wonders of science.

■

■

What a piece of work is a man!

—William Shakespeare, in *Hamlet*

■

CONTENTS

Contents ■9■

INTRODUCTION

■ Men have always been fascinated by their genitals, and this fascination begins at an early age. One of my gynecology colleagues insists he can tell the sex of a fetus instantly when the mother comes in for an ultrasound. "If I see the hands near the crotch, I know it's a boy," he jokes.

Despite this precocious interest, most men are woefully ignorant about the how and why of their reproductive organs. I will never forget the Harvard professor who consulted with me early in my career about a vasectomy. "I know it's a fairly simple procedure," he said, "but you're going to have to explain to me what is connected to what down there. I'm afraid I just never understood how that part of my body is put together."

The consequences of being ignorant about how the male organs operate may be considerable. A man who is relatively uninformed about an operation on his penis for impotence, for instance, may have unrealistic expectations for the surgery, which can lead to a major disappointment even though the surgeon considers the procedure a complete success. Some men believe (incorrectly) that awakening once a night to urinate is a sure sign of prostate cancer, and they worry for months before they finally find the courage to see their doctor.

There may be a significant psychological toll in other ways as well. I have seen many completely normal men in their twenties and thirties who feel terrible about themselves because they do not perform sexually the way they think they should, based on what they see in erotic movies, or from inflated stories of sexual athletics described over a few drinks. Although reassurance and education about what constitutes normal sexual behavior go a long way toward helping these men, in many cases the scars run deep, and a man's self-image may already have been seriously damaged by growing up informed by myths rather than knowledge.

The problem of poor general information about male reproductive biology is compounded by a lack of available written material on the subject. A search through the "health" or "men's" section of your local bookstore is likely to yield numerous volumes on diet, exercise, cholesterol, and your heart, but nothing on how to do a self-examination of the testicles to detect possible early tumors, or what to do if you are having sexual difficulties.

Women moved out of the sexual Dark Ages partly by writing and having access to books, such as *Our Bodies, Ourselves*, that included descriptions of the female reproductive system as well as aspects of normal sexuality in a clear, nonjudgmental way. The men's movement is now upon us, twenty years behind the women's movement. Men are now approaching their maleness with pride, much as women rejoiced in their female qualities beginning in the seventies. And just as women took strength from learning about their special biology, so, too, should men now learn about their unique inner workings.

The current hunger for information for and about men prompted me to write this book. As director of the Male Infertility and Impotence Program at Beth Israel Hospital, Harvard Medical School, in Boston, I see a wide variety of men with problems related to their genitals. A large part of my time with patients is devoted to educating them about their prostates, penises, and testicles. Many of these men are having difficulty fathering children or are unable to achieve adequate erections or have trouble urinating. Some may be concerned about the size or appearance of their penis, and others may be worried about the possibility of cancer in the testis or prostate.

Some new treatments are now available for many of these problems that may not be known to those outside the medical community. Indeed, many physicians may be unaware of some of these since the field is moving forward so rapidly. In these pages I describe these new developments as well as the standard treatments, with an occasional glimpse into the future. As a researcher, I hope also to share some of my enthusiasm for learning about how the body works.

Rather than presenting the information in a textbook manner, I have described actual cases from my practice that illustrate the problems and concerns from a more personal perspective. Names and many of the details of these cases have been changed to preserve the confidentiality of my patients. In some instances I have combined information from two or more cases to highlight an issue.

The book is divided into two main sections. Part I describes the normal events within the womb that cause a fetus to be born as a boy, followed by what takes place normally with male reproduction and with urination. The second section is devoted to problem areas and their treatment, primarily infertility, impotence, and prostate or urination problems.

If you have picked up this book to learn more about a specific problem, I recommend that you first read through the pertinent section on normal functioning in Part I before moving on to the appropriate segments in Part II. If you are under the care of a doctor, remember that individual considerations greatly influence what kind of treatment may be appropriate for you. This book contains my personal opinions, and other physicians may not agree with all of them. Treatments outlined here should be considered suggestions rather than rules, and they in no way substitute for the recommendations of your own physician, who knows you best.

This book is intended for men of all ages, although I hope that women with a curiosity about the human body in its various forms will be interested as well. My main goal has been to bring into the light a broad subject often cloaked in myth and misinformation. Although the male reproductive organs are never seen in public and are rarely discussed, the issues of sex, sexuality, and reproduction are part of our daily lives and elicit frequent responses from us, conscious or otherwise. For some men these responses are profound, particularly for those struggling with infertility or sexual inadequacy. Discussing these subjects openly in this book may be an opportunity for men and women to think about the male condition with more clarity and insight. If knowledge is power, then self-knowledge is empowering. I hope you enjoy reading this book as much as I have enjoyed writing it.

PART I

Where, what, how, when, and why

CHAPTER 1

DEVELOPMENT

■ IT'S A BOY!

A fetus develops into a male child in an amazing sequence of events that require precise coordination and chemical controls. Sometimes nature's quirks produce abnormal situations that help us understand normal development.

A young South American man named Luis came to my office shortly after arriving in the United States. Luis was born with a scrotum but without testicles. Doctors had told Luis's mother that there was nothing to be done. As an adolescent, Luis was again told by his local doctor that he would simply have to live his life with an empty scrotum. Now twenty-one, he wanted to be "normal."

With Luis's brother acting as an interpreter, I learned several important things. Luis had gone through puberty at the same time as his classmates, he was able to have firm erections, and he had engaged in intercourse on several occasions. Although his

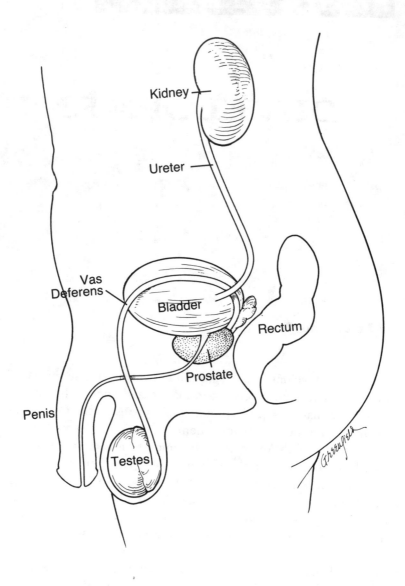

The male genital and urinary structures are illustrated from the side.

interest in sex, or libido, was strong, Luis refrained from sexual activity because ejaculation caused him to have pain deep in his pelvis. The main issue, however, was that Luis did not feel complete as a man, and this inhibited him from meeting women and considering marriage.

Luis was thin but muscular and had a nicely trimmed beard. He certainly looked like a normal young man with his pants on. However, when I examined Luis's scrotum, it was very small and tight, and I could not feel any testicles. I examined his groins carefully, since the testicles can occasionally become stuck in this region as they make their way to the scrotum during the last month or so in the womb. No testicles were felt in the groin either. Blood tests showed Luis had normal levels of testosterone, a hormone made by the testicles, so they had to be somewhere. A sophisticated X ray called a CT scan showed that his testicles were in his pelvis.

After discussion with Luis and his brother, we agreed to operate. My goal was to bring one or both of the testes down into the scrotum if possible. The limitation might be how healthy the testes appeared, and whether the blood vessels would be long enough to reach to the scrotum. Initially I was pleased to find the testicles low in the abdomen, appearing quite healthy. To my surprise, however, a thick-walled tubular structure between the testes extended down behind the pubic bone. Attached to this unusual structure were two armlike projections that stretched out to the testes. The tubular structure turned out to be a uterus, and the projections attached to the testes were fallopian tubes, which in the female carry the eggs from the ovary to the uterus. I removed the uterus and was able to bring one testicle into the scrotum but not the other.

Despite the presence of a uterus and fallopian tubes, Luis was indeed a man, but had a condition called male pseudohermaphroditism. True hermaphrodites have both a testicle and an ovary. Pseudohermaphrodites have some physical characteristics of the opposite sex, but have normal gonads (in this case testicles), although they may be in abnormal locations. Some pseudohermaphrodites have such a poorly developed penis and scrotum that they are mistaken at birth for females. Luis, however, had appeared completely normal at birth except for his missing testicles, and it was therefore quite a surprise to find internal female structures.

How could such an accident of nature take place? In order to answer this, it is necessary to understand normal sexual development. The information that determines whether a child will be blond or dark haired, male or female, is carried by the sperm and egg in packages of information called genes, which are made up of chemicals called DNA (deoxyribonucleic acid). DNA appears in each mammalian cell as a number of long strands called chromosomes, with each chromosome carrying the information of hundreds to thousands of genes. Animals have different numbers of chromosomes, with humans having twenty-three pairs, forty-six overall. One of these pairs is called the sex chromosomes because they carry genes that determine the sex of the offspring. Chromosomes are usually examined at a time when they look like the letter X. The chromosome that carries the information to make a boy, however, is shorter and is called the Y chromosome. A human male, therefore, has a set of chromosomes described as 46 XY.

The Y chromosome has a special function in the developing fetus to direct sexual differentiation. At seven weeks, the human fetus has a gonad (the general term for either testis or ovary), and primitive tubular structures that are undifferentiated, that is, they are neither male nor female. By the eighth week, under the influence of the Y chromosome, the gonad begins to produce two chemicals that will ultimately cause masculinization of the genital structures.

The first of these is testosterone, a steroid hormone that is often called the "male" hormone, since it is produced almost exclusively by the testis. Testosterone causes the undifferentiated tubes to become the vas deferens and the epididymis, which in the adult male carry sperm from the testis to the penis. Testosterone is also converted to a second hormone, dihydrotestosterone (DHT), which acts to masculinize the penis and scrotum. Without these hormones, the scrotum forms instead as the labia majora, or outer lips of the vagina, and the penis is tiny and indistinguishable from the female clitoris.

Another remarkable story of abnormal development that aids our understanding of the normal process of sexual differentiation occurs among an inbred group in the Dominican Republic. This group has a high incidence of a genetic defect that results in the absence of the enzyme needed to convert testosterone to DHT. As a result, some of these male infants are born with female external genitalia, namely, with a vagina, labia, and a small phallic structure that more closely resembles a clitoris than a penis. They are indistinguishable from normal girls at birth and are raised as girls. Remarkably, at puberty, the testicles begin to produce such large amounts of testosterone that masculinization occurs, with appearance of a beard, lowering of the voice, and penile growth. These individuals abandon their skirts and begin to wear pants. The chromosomes of these individuals are 46 X, Y, just as for other males.

As remarkable as the biological changes that occur in these boys is the ease with which they are accepted into their society. No stigma is attached to them. It is simply understood among these people that a small number of the little girls playing among themselves will one day turn out to be boys, who will then work and play with the rest of the men. In contrast, when there is doubt about the true sex of a child born with ambiguous genitalia in the United States, it is considered a medical and social emergency. Parents in our culture have tremendous difficulty coping with uncertainty about their child's future development. We need to know whether our newborn child is a boy or a girl. Exploratory surgery and extensive X rays may be carried out in the first days of life to identify what internal structures are present.

In some cases a very difficult decision is made by parents and doctors to raise a child as the opposite sex from what the chromosomes intended. For example, a boy may be born with two undescended testicles, like Luis, and may in addition have a scrotum split down the middle like a girl's labia, together with a tiny, poorly developed penis. This child's genitalia could never look normal as a male's, but with surgery it is likely that a fairly normal female appearance could be created. In terms of self-image and group acceptance, this appears to be of paramount importance. This is an excruciatingly difficult process for parents, yet it seems to work out just fine as long as decisions are made very early in life.

The second substance produced by the developing testis is called müllerian inhibiting substance (MIS). The early internal tubular structures that in the female become the uterus, fallopian tubes, and part of the vagina are called müllerian ducts. In the normal male, these structures disappear under the influence of MIS. If one testis fails to form properly within the male fetus, a partially developed uterus and fallopian tube will be found on that side. Again, in the absence of direction from the testis, the internal and external genital structures of an individual will develop as female.

Given this background, how does one explain what happened to Luis? His testosterone levels were normal and both testicles were present, yet he had müllerian duct structures, which are normally found in a woman, but which should regress and disappear in a man. Two possibilities exist: either his testicles failed to produce MIS at the critical period when the müllerian ducts should have been told to disappear, or the müllerian ducts did not recognize MIS and continued to develop as if no testicles were present. Through sophisticated laboratory analysis Luis's blood was found to contain normal amounts of MIS for his age. Presumably it was also present twenty-one years previously. The most likely explanation is that the uterus and fallopian tubes lacked the chemical ability to recognize MIS, and they therefore did not disappear as they should have done.

What about the undescended testicles? How does that happen? During development, the cells that make up the testicle migrate from an area near the spinal column to form a gonad complete with a tough capsule around it called the tunica albug-inea. The developing testis at this point lies internally, near the level of the kidney, and its blood and nerve supply arise from nearby structures. Over the next several months the testis descends into the lower part of the abdomen, and during the eighth month it passes through a hole in the abdominal wall called the inguinal canal to take up its final position in the scrotum. The area around the inguinal canal is often called the groin, and it lies just above and parallel to the skin crease dividing the thigh from the torso.

On its way through the inguinal canal the testis becomes wrapped by the lining of the abdominal cavity (the peritoneum), and occasionally a loop of intestine may follow the path of the testis, creating an unhappy bulge in the groin or scrotum. This is called a hernia. When the doctor sticks his finger up the scrotum into the groin and gives the famous instructions to "turn your head and cough," he is feeling for a bulge in the groin that indicates a hernia.

What tells the testis to make this incredible journey? A fibrous band attaches to the lower part of the testicle at one end, and to the scrotum on the other end, and appears essentially to "pull" the testis along its downward course. Approximately one out of a hundred times the testis fails to descend normally on one or both sides. This is called cryptorchidism, which literally means "hidden testis." The testis may get hung up anywhere along the way, such as near the kidneys, in the pelvis, or most commonly within the inguinal canal. Rarely, it can take a wrong turn and end up in front of the pubic bone or behind the scrotum.

After losing touch with Luis for nearly a year, I received a call from a young man speaking nearly perfect English. To my amazement, it was Luis. He subsequently came into the office with a big smile on his face. The right testicle was in the scrotum, small but adequate. He was sexually active and quite pleased with himself and his new life in the United States. Although artificial testicles made of silicone provide an excellent cosmetic appearance for men missing a testis, Luis was not at all interested in this. As far as he was concerned, he had one testis more than when he had started, and that was enough. He now felt like a man. The pain with ejaculation had disappeared as well. Although I cannot be sure, I suspect this pain may have been due to secretion of semen into his uterus, where a normal semen chemical called prostaglandin may have caused strong uterine contractions. With removal of the uterus, the pain had resolved.

When I presented Luis's case at a medical conference, I was asked what I had told him about the surgical findings, in particular what I had said about the uterus and fallopian tubes. This really brings up the issue of what is the proper role of a physician. My philosophy as a physician is to provide as complete information as possible to my patients. However, one of the challenges and responsibilities of a physician is to be able to speak about delicate issues in delicate terms. Often this means avoiding emotionally loaded words or phrases. This may be particularly difficult when there is a language barrier.

I felt that Luis had a right to know what I had found, but I also did not want to tell him something that could be misconstrued by him, or by his brother doing the translating, to indicate that Luis was some kind of freak. I therefore told him that I had removed certain structures that should have disappeared early in development.

In the year since I had last seen him, Luis had found a job as a grocery clerk and had learned English by taking night classes. The quiet, shy man I had first met was now outgoing, happy, and quite a talker. He had applied to college and was hoping to stay in the United States.

A clue as to what it meant for Luis to have a testicle was provided by a gift he gave me, sent from his home. Luis came to my office and brought out two delicate, carefully wrapped objects. As he removed the wrapping, I thought he was presenting me with two enormous porcelain or china testicles, the size of a grapefruit. In fact, they were ostrich eggs, the largest eggs in the world, and an item of some value. I could not help but wonder whether the gift to me of this reproductive trophy reflected Luis's new sense of his own virility.

When a healthy male infant is born, the doctor glances at the genitals and does not hesitate to announce "It's a boy!" The plain fact of a normal penis and scrotum appearing in their expected locations does not usually generate much appreciation for the wonders of human development. However, the more one learns, the clearer it becomes that the birth of a little boy or girl is a true marvel of nature.

■ PUBERTY

After a brief period of activity during fetal life when testosterone helps mold the developing baby into a boy, the testicles go into a state of suspended animation, like being put into the deep freeze. They make very little testosterone and no sperm. This quiet period ends with a time of life we call puberty. *Puber* is actually Latin for adulthood. At this time, the brain receives some signal, as yet unknown, and begins to put its part of the sleeping hormonal machinery into action. Hormones are chemicals made by one part of the body but whose actions take place elsewhere, often at distant sites. Hormones were first noted for their stimulatory functions, as in hyperthyroidism, due to excess thyroid hormone, which causes the metabolism to speed up. They therefore took their name from the Greek *horman*, meaning to urge on.

The hypothalamus, situated deep within the substance of the brain, controls many of the basic functions of life. In this part of the brain are control centers for hunger and thirst, temperature regulation, sexual activity, and sleep. The hypothalamus is also a production center for hormones that affect many distant locations within the body.

For design reasons not yet understood by mortals, the hypothalamus tends to exert its hormonal influence indirectly, through another part of the brain called the pituitary. The pituitary hangs down from the base of the brain on a little stalk, like a cherry at the tip of a stem. Along the stem runs a short blood highway carrying hormones from the hypothalamus. In response to hypothalamic signals, the pituitary produces and releases a variety of hormones into the circulatory system, some of which travel to the testicles.

When the puberty alarm clock goes off, the hypothalamus begins to send signals to the pituitary to release large amounts of hormones called luteinizing hormone (LH) and follicle-stimulating hormone (FSH). These same hormones are released during female puberty, but act somewhat differently in women. LH and FSH travel through the bloodstream to act on the testes. FSH works directly on the Sertoli cells within the seminiferous tubules, and LH stimulates the Leydig cells, which lie in the spaces between tubules and are responsible for the production of testosterone.

FSH seems critical for the Sertoli cells to get into gear and create the proper environment for sperm development, although the details are scarcely known. The effect of LH is somewhat better understood, presumably because its actions can be more easily dissected chemically. As far as we know, the action of the Leydig cell is to make testosterone, period. It makes testosterone only under the proper circumstances, namely when there are adequate amounts of LH present. The Leydig cell is very hardy and withstands high temperatures and even radiation without too much trouble.

Testosterone is made from cholesterol, which is abundantly present in blood and enters the Leydig cell as its raw material. In a series of enzymatic steps, chemical pieces are added and removed from cholesterol to form testosterone. Once made, testosterone is released from the Leydig cell, free either to enter the bloodstream or to be trapped by molecules within the Sertoli cell.

It is no coincidence that the Leydig cells are located in the testes, next door to the seminiferous tubules. The testes have the highest concentration of testosterone in the body as a result of this. Testosterone is so important to the developing germ cells that the Sertoli cell manufactures a special protein whose job is to latch onto testosterone molecules and carry it around to all levels of the developing germ cells. It is the high level of testosterone within the testes that finally allows sperm development to occur, although the high adult FSH levels are critical as well. The high testosterone level results in what we more readily recognize as the signs of male puberty.

Testosterone or the related hormone dihydrotestosterone (DHT) stimulates increased hair growth, particularly in the pubic region, and soon afterward in the beard. Hair in the armpits appears, to the gratitude of deodorant manufacturers. The larynx, or voice box, enlarges, creating a prominent Adam's apple and lower vocal pitch. Muscular definition appears. The penis and testicles undergo a period of growth, the latter primarily due to the increased activity and presence of more numerous germ cells at all levels of development. Even the bones of the body respond to testosterone, accounting in part for the growth spurt of adolescence. Finally, there are emotional and mental changes resulting from the influence of testosterone on the brain, such as an awareness of sexuality and sexual urges.

These changes are so remarkable, and occur over such a short period of time, that it is easy to understand the awkwardness of the adolescent male. After all, who he is today seems already so different from who he was even a few days ago.

CHAPTER 2

THE PENIS

■ The preoccupation of men with the size of their penis and the competitive instincts that surround it are typified in this story told to me by a patient. Three men walk out of a bar in a small town and stop on a small bridge to empty their bladders. They lean out over the edge in the dark and begin to urinate. The first man says, "River sure is cold." The second man says, "It's deep, too." The third man says, "Sandy bottom."

Although the testicles are arguably more important in determining maleness, the penis is generally considered the main structure that distinguishes men from women. Certainly, as little boys and girls examine their naked bodies and compare them, it is the penis that stands out as the organ of contention. Freud's theories on female psychology, now largely considered flawed and of historical interest only, were based on the concept of penis envy, i.e., that women lacked a critical organ denoting power and dominance and sought to make up for this loss or emptiness by misdirected emotional means. Current psychological thought sees other motivational factors influencing female development. Yet there is little question that

Freud's emphasis on the psychological importance of the penis was correct, at least for men.

Men spend a great deal of time thinking about their penis for one reason or another. It serves as a sexual organ and as an organ of urination. The size is often felt to be an indicator of one's sexuality and desirability. The penis has also been used as an emblem of one's religious background. It follows, then, that problems with the penis can cause tremendous consternation for the owner. The privacy surrounding the penis, rarely referred to by its proper name in public, leads to a mythology with little relation to reality. In the following pages I shall attempt to shed some light on this fascinating organ.

■ DEVELOPMENT AND ANATOMY OF THE PENIS

The penis develops in the embryo from a small mound of tissue that also forms the clitoris in the female. It consists of two erectile cylinders called the corpora cavernosa (cavernous bodies), which fill with blood during erection, as well as a third cylinder called the corpus spongiosum (spongy body). The corpus spongiosum includes the urethra, which is the tube leading from the bladder to the tip of the penis. As the corpus spongiosum reaches the tip of the penis, it flares out to form the head of the penis, which sits like a mushroom cap atop the two corpora cavernosa.

One of the more common things that can go awry with the penis is generally diagnosed during early childhood. Jimmy was two years old when his father noticed that Jimmy's penis was bent downward whenever he had an erection. Jimmy never seemed to complain about this and appeared to urinate freely, although Jimmy's dad wondered whether the urine was coming from a spot somewhere along the shaft rather than from the tip. Jimmy was otherwise a perfectly healthy boy with a healthy older sister.

On examination Jimmy was a robust, active two-year-old,

with a normal abdomen, normal testicles, and on first inspection a fairly normal penis. However, on closer examination the foreskin was incompletely formed around the bottom, so that the skin on the top surface looked more like a hood. On lifting the penis up, the opening in the urethra was on the bottom surface of the shaft of the penis just behind the head, or glans. Additionally, by pushing down on the skin and fat on either side of the penis in order to make it protrude more, there appeared to be a downward tilt to the head of the penis, beginning at the point where the urethra opened.

What was wrong with Jimmy? The medical term is *hypospadias*, which resulted from incomplete development of the urethra and associated tissues. The urethra forms normally by infolding of skin along the bottom of the penis, creating a tube that is later covered by skin. Except for the very tip of the penis where it appears in the center of the glans, the urethra runs just below the skin on the bottom of the penis and can be felt there as a soft, spongy, collapsed tube. In Jimmy's case, the infolding of skin never took place along the farthest part of the penis, so that the tube stopped before it reached the end. This didn't interfere with Jimmy's urinating because the penile urethra acts only as a conduit for the urine flow and helps to direct it. Water will continue to come out of a hose even if you remove a segment at the end.

For reasons that are unclear, in hypospadias the penile skin fails to form a normal foreskin in the area of the shortened urethra, so that a hood occurs rather than the circumferential foreskin. Finally, some boys with hypospadias develop what is essentially scar tissue from the vicinity of the urethral opening all the way out to the tip of the penis. This scar tissue, called chordee, causes the downward curvature of the penis with an erection.

Think of the penis as a cylindrical balloon. If you placed a piece of tape along a portion of the balloon and then inflated it, it would curve toward the side with the tape, since the taped portion would be unable to expand as much as the rest of the balloon. Scar tissue in the penis causes the same problem.

Hypospadias occurs in mild and severe forms, depending on how far the opening is from the tip and the degree of chordee. When it is severe, the opening may be at the junction of the penis and the scrotum, or even behind the scrotum. In its mildest form the opening may be just short of the center of the glans, noticeable only to an experienced physician or urologist. This minor form of hypospadias often goes untreated without any consequences. Otherwise, hypospadias is important to treat, and to treat early. Not only does the ability to properly direct the urinary stream become more important as boys outgrow their diapers but the bent penis may also interfere with normal sexual functioning. Equally important is the impact of an odd-looking penis on a boy's sense of self as he reaches puberty, particularly on his fragile sense of sexual identity.

Hypospadias is treated surgically by creating a tube from skin or other body tissues to bridge the gap between the existing hole and the tip of the penis. Often, as the scar tissue of chordee is removed and the underside of the penis is freed up, the actual gap is found to be much greater than was apparent preoperatively, when the penis was still tethered. Boys with mild forms of hypospadias are treated as outpatients, whereas more extensive hypospadias surgery may require a hospital stay of several days up to a week. Since surgery can be technically difficult, it should generally be performed by an experienced pediatric urologist. Results are usually quite good cosmetically and functionally.

Jimmy's parents agreed to have his hypospadias corrected surgically. At surgery, an artificial erection was created by filling the penis under pressure with fluid. This demonstrated a severe bend to the tip of the penis. After careful removal of the scar tissue, the head of the penis stood straight up. However, the gap between the urethral opening and the tip of the penis was now much greater. Jimmy's hood of foreskin was removed, rolled into a tube, was stitched at one end to the existing urethral opening, and at the other end was brought up through the glans to form an opening at the tip of the penis. The skin of the penis was then used to cover the new tube. The appearance was excellent, and Jimmy urinated through the tip of his penis for the first time in his life.

For those who doubt the emotional significance of having a penis that differs from what we consider normal, there is the sobering example of epispadias. This is a rare condition in which the penis is flattened and shortened with the urine opening being just above the junction of the penis and the skin above. The penis looks like a spade, or like a hot dog that has been scored lengthwise. There is no urethral tube, just a furrow where the urine drains constantly. Frequently this condition coexists with a bladder lying on the surface of the abdomen, called exstrophy. The superficial bladder is usually repaired and placed within the abdomen within the first days to weeks of life. The penis, however, may not be repaired until much later.

The suicide rate for adolescent boys with epispadias had been extremely high in the past, as they struggled with their deficient sexual body image at a time when minute details of appearance play a tremendous role in self-esteem. If a facial pimple is enough for many teenagers to feel embarrassed and awkward in social situations, one can only imagine what it feels like to be an adolescent with a terribly misshapen penis. Fortunately, surgery can be performed to make these penises look quite acceptable.

■ SIZE

One of the most common things men worry about is the size of their penis. Somehow the idea of being "well hung" has permeated our civilization as the quintessential feature of the desirable male. The appearance of particularly well-endowed men in erotic movies and magazines has certainly added to the mistaken belief among many men, especially those who have had little opportunity to see other men naked, that a penis of eight inches or more is the norm. The corollary seems to be that a smaller penis is inadequate.

This emphasis on size is not peculiar to Western culture in the late twentieth century. As of several years ago, it was possible to pay a few extra dollars upon visiting the restored Roman ruins at Pompeii from A.D. 79 to see a fresco of a wealthy man using his enormous penis to counterbalance several bags of money on an ancient scale. Clearly, the message is that a large phallus is worth its weight in gold. The problem in today's world is that men with perfectly normal penises feel inadequate and are afraid to meet women because of the risk of humiliation. Where does this concern come from?

Psychologists argue that the focus on penis size stems from early comparisons with one's father. A child's penis is indeed a small organ, although it does become erect quite regularly. This does not indicate sexual arousal nor a history of sexual awareness or abuse, as some parents have feared. During puberty, as the testes begin to produce large amounts of testosterone, the penis begins to grow considerably in length and girth. This accompanies some of the other changes occurring at that time, such as the appearance of facial hair and deepening of the voice. As the child looks to his father as his rival for his mother's affections, so the theory goes, he is constantly comparing himself, "sizing" himself up next to his father.

The competitive spirit that this engenders is felt to be quite adaptive as a motivating force to the young boy, and as he grows older and finds that in many ways he has equaled his father, this results in a sense of accomplishment, satisfaction, and self-worth. In terms of sexuality, of assessing one's attractiveness, the period of competition for mother occurs primarily at a time when the boy is hopelessly unequal to his father in a physical sense. As the boy grows older and his penis enlarges as well, the competition for mother changes. Girls his own age become the main objects of his affection. In effect, the game changes before the growing boy actually achieves some degree of equality with his father in terms of penis size.

When a patient brings up concerns about the size of his penis, I like to tell them the story of Abraham Lincoln. President Lincoln was extremely tall for his time and was once asked his opinion on the proper length of a man's legs. His commonsense answer was that a man's legs should be long enough to reach from his hips to the ground. In similar fashion, a man's penis should be long enough to reach inside his partner. For this is the essential biological function of a penis in the first place, to enter the vagina so that semen is deposited near the opening of the uterus, called the cervix. A larger penis does not necessarily perform this task better than a smaller penis.

Despite these comments, patients will still usually ask, "Well, what is the length of a normal penis?" The problem with giving numbers is that people automatically run to their tape measure to see how they measure up, which defeats the purpose of what I have been trying to say. Namely, if a man has been able to have satisfactory intercourse, then his penis is just fine.

Of course, one of the most remarkable things about a penis is how it changes size during the course of every day. During moments of anxiety or when a man is cold, the penis shrinks up. When feeling comfortable or warm, it will fill up like a water balloon, even without sexual arousal. For the record, the flaccid penis generally ranges from three to six inches and enlarges by approximately two inches in length when erect.

Actually, the penis is considerably longer than people realize. Normally men think of their penis as extending from the tip of the glans to the pubic bone. However, what most men do not appreciate is that the penis continues beneath the scrotal sac and ends nearly at the base of the bone in the seat. As the penile cylinders make their way beneath the scrotum, they fan out like the arms of the letter Y and attach themselves to the bones connecting the pubic bone to the bone at the base of the buttocks. This anchors the penis so that when it is rigid, it does not simply wave in the breeze. Penetration would be a difficult matter without this bony anchor. Large mammals such as the walrus require even more help, in the form of a bone or cartilage called

a baculum, which extends along the length of the penis below
the skin to provide adequate support for intercourse.

A patient of mine called one day to ask if I would be willing
to see his twenty-five-year-old son. His son was a "good kid"
who had had one testicle removed as a child because it had not
descended, and who also had concerns that his penis was small.
As a result of this, he was afraid to meet girls, kept to himself,
had few male friends, and stayed home with his parents.

When I met Charlie, he seemed like a pleasant young man.
He told me that he had had an experience five years earlier
where a girl he knew only slightly had made fun of him during a
sexual encounter, commenting that his penis was small. He had
not had another sexual encounter since then. Charlie had also
seen some X-rated movies and felt that his penis just did not
measure up to those of the men in the movies. Finally, he had
some concerns about having just one testicle. Did this mean he
was somehow less virile, less potent?

In effect, Charlie was wondering whether he was much of a
man. He had a good job and, apart from his lack of sociability,
led a normal life. He was likable and nice looking. On examination, Charlie had a good physique as he kept himself in shape.
A normal amount of body hair and muscle definition indicated
that Charlie's remaining testicle was producing sufficient levels
of testosterone. His penis was of average length and girth. One
testis was absent, and the other was completely normal.

It seemed to me that the most important things I could offer
Charlie were information about his genitals and my perspective
on his situation. I told him the size of his penis was normal. The
absent testicle placed him among a large group of men who had
lost a testicle due to trauma, infection, or cryptorchidism, and
the vast majority of these men had normal sex lives and families.
His testosterone levels could be checked with a blood test, but
I had no doubt they were normal. The absent testis did not affect
the size of his penis or his fertility. An artificial testicle called a
prosthesis could be inserted in his scrotum if he wished. Finally,
the sarcastic comment made by the girl years ago was cruel and

insensitive and probably reflected her own sexual insecurities. Certainly she had no feelings for Charlie, and so she had been a poor choice with whom to share an intimate event.

Charlie listened quietly to what I had to say and left the office. I never heard from him again. A year later, though, I saw Charlie's father back in the office. As he was leaving, he said, "Thank you so much for all you did for Charlie. He's like a new person." Soon after his visit to me, Charlie had started going out in the evening with friends from work. He met a girl and was dating her on a regular basis. He moved into his own apartment. According to his father, Charlie had just "opened up like a flower."

I take a great deal of satisfaction from my experience with Charlie. I suspect Charlie would have come to the same point without ever seeing me, but I like to think I played some role in helping him along. It was not the usual doctor-patient interaction. There was no illness, I provided no diagnosis and no treatment. And yet I think of Charlie as one of my greatest successes. I learned a lot from Charlie as well, specifically about the fragile nature of the male ego. What a man does depends on how he sees himself, and how he sees himself may be determined by perceptions (correct or false) of his sexual adequacy. By helping Charlie readjust some of his thoughts and self-perceptions, he was able to move forward emotionally and learn to interact successfully in the social world. There are so many differences between people that it is easy to lose sight of how broad a category is defined by the term *normal*.

■ THE FORESKIN—TO HAVE OR HAVE NOT

John walked into my office requesting a circumcision. A twenty-two-year-old man with a steady girlfriend, he complained that after sex he would develop cuts and bruises on his penis, confined for the most part to the foreskin. On examination I saw that he had an uncircumcised penis with small bruises and lacerations around the foreskin. This was a fairly unusual complaint, and I wondered whether John was particularly energetic during intercourse or engaged in anal intercourse without adequate lubrication. His own impression was that the injuries resulted from the back-and-forth movement of his foreskin during intercourse. Hence, his desire to have the foreskin removed.

Circumcision in the newborn is common in the United States and is generally performed within a few minutes and without anesthesia. In the older child and adult, however, it is a more significant procedure, requiring some form of anesthesia, and taking thirty to forty-five minutes to perform. There is a small risk of bleeding and infection. I therefore like to be sure that there is a good reason to operate before I perform a circumcision, and I was not convinced that John's problem would be solved by surgery.

I told John that the solution to his problem was to use lubrication such as petroleum jelly (but not with condoms, which can be dissolved by this) or a water-soluble lubricant (no problem for condoms), and to call me in a month if things were no better. A month later John reported that the bruising on the foreskin was only slightly better, and the lacerations persisted. He had increased the amount of lubrication to the point that he could hardly feel any penile stimulation during intercourse. Again he asked me to perform a circumcision. After cautioning John that his bruising might persist even after his circumcision, I agreed. Under general anesthesia, the foreskin was removed and the skin was sutured together. John was now circumcised. He went home several hours later and healed nicely. Two months after John had resumed sexual activity, he returned to see me. "Doc, the bruising and cuts are completely gone. I told you this was what I needed!"

The foreskin is a specialized piece of skin that arises from the shaft of the penis, extends outward, and folds back on itself in such a way as to sheathe the glans. Some men have foreskins that completely cover the glans, making it invisible unless the foreskin is retracted, and others are born with only a rudimentary extra flap of skin so that the entire glans is visible except for the rim, called the corona, meaning crown. The function of the foreskin is not known, although one could argue that it serves to protect the sensitive glans.

Over the ages, circumcision was reserved for ritual or religious purposes. In the Jewish faith, the circumcision is performed on the eighth day of life by a specially trained religious person, the mohel, in a celebration called a briss. At that time the child receives his Hebrew name and is officially welcomed into the community. Moslems perform circumcision later in life, as a ritual welcoming of the child into manhood.

The push to perform widespread newborn circumcisions in this country began after World War II, carried along by new attitudes of cleanliness and sanitation. The medical community believed that the circumcised penis was easier to clean and less prone to infection. There also came reports that cancer of the penis occurred almost exclusively among uncircumcised men, so that circumcision became a protective measure against that terrible disease. Medical attitudes became public policy, and a majority of newborn males have been circumcised in the United States from the 1950s to the present.

In the 1980s there was a backlash of public and medical opinion regarding the merits of routine circumcision. Emphasis on the baby's pain weighed against the minor risks of being uncircumcised in a relatively clean society created a confusing picture for parents of newborn boys. Although it is true that penile cancer occurs primarily in uncircumcised men, the incidence of this disease in the United States is so small even among uncircumcised men that it is hard to justify circumcision on that basis. In the last few years, however, there has again been a swing back to circumcision, as it appears that infant boys who are circumcised are less apt to get bladder infections than those who are not.

Does this mean that circumcisions should be routinely performed? My own feeling is that where there is no religious or cultural reason for the circumcision, parents should do what they feel most comfortable with. In this country there seems to be no lasting physical or emotional problem that results either from having or not having a foreskin. I consider it a matter of personal choice.

What is the difference between a circumcised and uncircumcised penis? Very little, really. Men who undergo an adult circumcision usually describe an increased sensitivity to the head of the penis, which may bother them for a month or so as their underwear rubs against the penis. The circumcised penis is slightly easier to keep clean, since there is no need to retract the foreskin during bathing. However, these are minor issues. The main difference is how the penis looks.

It is important for uncircumcised men to retract the foreskin at least once daily to wash, and generally with each urination. If the foreskin is never retracted, it is easy to develop infections underneath, particularly yeast infections. When this occurs, the glans becomes red and inflamed, and there is usually a creamy or cheesy discharge. Infections may also lead to scarring of the foreskin so that the opening becomes so tight that the foreskin cannot be retracted at all. This condition, called phimosis, is the most common reason for performing an adult circumcision. Diabetics seem to be at higher risk for developing infections under the foreskin, often requiring a circumcision to prevent recurrences.

■ ERECTIONS

The penis has three functions: to direct the urinary stream, to become rigid enough to allow penetration during intercourse, and to deposit semen within the vagina during ejaculation. For the first and third of these, the penis acts essentially as a passive conduit, with the urethra serving as the pipeline. However, the middle function, that of achieving an erection, is a remarkable piece of engineering unique to the penis that requires an active process.

The penis is composed of three cylinders. One cylinder is the corpus spongiosum, which contains the urethra and blood vessels, and the other two are the paired corpora cavernosa. The corpora cavernosa are responsible for developing rigidity and are thus called the erectile bodies. As we have seen previously, the corpora cavernosa extend from the tip of the penis just behind the glans, through the shaft of the penis, underneath the scrotal sac, and down each side of the bone connecting the pubic bone to the bone at the base of the buttocks, upon which we sit.

A central artery runs down the middle of each corpus cavernosa. Blood from the artery enters the spongy tissue of the penis, which is lined by muscle. The blood leaves the corpora cavernosa through small veins that run obliquely through the tough sheath enveloping the corpora cavernosa. As the blood leaves the corpora cavernosa, it enters larger veins running around the penis from bottom to top, finally entering the main vein draining the penis, called the deep dorsal vein. This runs along the top surface of the penis from the glans to the pubic bone, where it dives underneath. Many men have one or several prominent veins visible just under the skin of the penis, which become engorged with an erection. These superficial veins drain the skin and glans of the penis, but not the corpora cavernosa. Arteries also run along the top surface of the penis, and a small pulse can often be felt in these. These superficial arteries provide nourishment to the skin and glans, but are also not involved in erections.

In the flaccid state, the blood requirement of the penis is small, and flow is minimal. The nerves governing the flaccid condition are called the sympathetic nerves, which are also the nerves releasing adrenaline during times of fear and anxiety. The effect of these nerves and the adrenaline they produce is to keep the muscle surrounding the arteries contracted. This keeps the diameter of the arteries small, and little blood flow occurs. Whatever blood makes it into the corpora cavernosa is free to flow right back out again.

During periods of sexual arousal, however, an opposing set of nerves, called the parasympathetic nerves, is stimulated. These

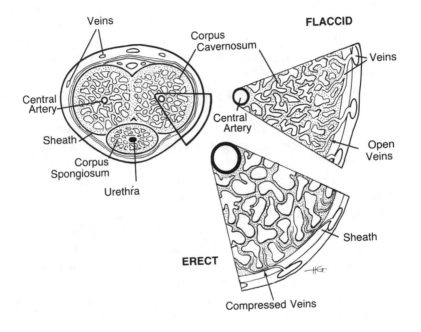

Cross section of the penis. The paired erectile chambers called the corpora cavernosa make up most of the bulk of the penis. The urethra is contained within the corpus spongiosum and runs along the underside of the penis until it reaches the glans, where it emerges in the center. The inset shows how the arteries and spongy tissue within the corpora cavernosa swell during erection, compressing the veins so that blood flow out of the penis is reduced.

nerves cause relaxation of the muscle around the arteries. The arteries expand, and blood flow into the corpora cavernosa increases dramatically. In order to create an erection the penis must not only allow increased filling but must also be able to trap the blood within it so that the erection can be maintained. Two events take place during arousal to produce this effect. First, the muscular lining around the spongy tissue within the corpora cavernosa relaxes, allowing blood to flow in with less resistance. Second, the veins running obliquely through the tough sheath are compressed, trapping blood within the corpora cavernosa. The internal pressure begins to rise, and the flow of blood into and out of the penis eventually slows to a trickle with a firm erection.

The sheath around the corpora cavernosa plays an interesting role in erection. It has some elasticity, which allows the penis to expand and shrink; however, its elasticity is fairly limited. This is a good thing, since infinite elasticity would result in enormous penises that would be completely useless, since the rigidity necessary for penetration would be missing. If a car tire or a football were as elastic as a balloon, it would not be functional; however, once it is completely stretched, each additional pump of air increases the internal pressure and it becomes firmer. Although the penis fills with blood rather than air, the same principle holds true. It is the limited stretch of the sheath around the corpora that confers rigidity to the penis.

If this is how an erection occurs, how does the penis soften? How does the blood escape from the penis? Why don't men walk around with perpetual erections? Again, it is the nerves that control what happens. After a man ejaculates or is distracted or loses his state of sexual arousal, the sympathetic nerves again come to the fore. Remember that they act in an opposite fashion to the parasympathetic nerves, which were responsible for creating the erection in the first place. The sympathetic nerves cause the arteries to close down, reducing the amount of blood that enters the penis. In addition, the spongy tissue holding the blood also contracts, relieving the compression on the veins against the sheath. Now blood can freely leave the corpora cavernosa, and soon the penis is flaccid.

Why do erections disappear following ejaculation? Ejaculation is a complex sequence of events, to be described in the next chapter, that is governed by the sympathetic nerves. As the climax occurs, there is a large discharge of adrenaline in the system. Flaccidity of the penis is one of the consequences of this discharge. For all men there is a period of time during which a second ejaculation cannot take place, and it may be difficult to immediately achieve another erection during this time as well. This is called the refractory period.

In young men the refractory period may be as short as several minutes. However, it lengthens with age, so that for most men beyond age forty it is at least twenty minutes and often much longer. Although the refractory period has not been studied in great depth in humans, it seems likely that it is related in part to overcoming the release of adrenaline that occurs with ejaculation. Changes within the sexual centers of the brain occur with ejaculation, and these centers must be reset before full sexual behavior can be produced. Clearly, the refractory period can be affected tremendously by the presence or absence of continued sexual arousal following ejaculation.

Sexual arousal is a complicated biological phenomenon. We recognize it by how it makes us feel, and we give it names such as being *turned on, aroused, horny,* or just *excited.* However, the actual events inside the body and brain are complicated. For younger men particularly, the sight, smell, sound, or touch of an attractive woman may be enough to initiate a sequence of events that results in an erection. Older men generally require physical stimulation to achieve a full erection. In the case of sight, what we see is light hitting the retinal nerves at the back of the eye. These nerves see only patterns of light, dark, and color, and they transmit this information to the back of the brain where the visual cortex processes the information and interprets it, for instance, as an attractive woman. Nerves from this center must then signal those parts of the brain involved in sexual behavior, and switches are turned on or off depending on what input arrives. The sexual center receives information from numerous sources, all of which modulate whether the final message that is put out is a state of arousal or not.

A situation that may be arousing under one set of circumstances may be completely nonsexual at other times, depending for example on fatigue, work, or stress. For some men, an exciting situation may be completely spoiled by one small detail, such as hearing the wrong type of music. The sexual center of the brain incorporates all this information on a moment-by-moment basis, and if all systems are "go," it sends a message via the parasympathetic nerves to the penis to begin erection. This message travels down the spinal cord to the lower part of the back, where the nerve exits and runs in the pelvis until it reaches the penis. If at the next moment the sexual center changes its mind, the sympathetic nerves are signaled, and the message runs down a similar course until the message reaches the penis and counteracts the first message.

Arousal is also influenced by how much time has elapsed since sex last occurred. Animal research can be helpful in evaluating the threshold at which sexual behavior is elicited, which is a reasonable way to investigate sexual arousal. The ringdove is typical of many animals in that it performs a complex ritual of movements and sounds directed to a receptive female as a prelude to actual intercourse. A male that has recently mated will perform this sexual dance only to females of the same species. After the male has been isolated for several days, however, he will perform this behavior in response to a wooden female dummy in his cage. With further isolation the behavior can be elicited by the dummy head alone. Eventually, the corners of the cage will be enough to provoke him to perform his sexual dance.

Most men can relate to this story about the ringdove. Men will universally admit that they become easily aroused if they have been unable to have sex for a long time. This degree of arousal can even be worrisome for some men, as they may feel consumed by their sexual interest. In the animal world, this is an easily understood adaptive process, since the drive to reproduce is extremely strong. And lest we forget, the biological reward for sex is reproduction.

CHAPTER 3

EJACULATION

■ Although we generally think of ejaculation and erection as being intimately associated with one another, they are actually two separate processes. Happily, they usually go together so well that we think of them as one event. The proof that ejaculation is not simply an extension of an erection is that when a man loses the ability to achieve an erection, he is still usually able to ejaculate.

Ejaculation is the body's way of bringing sperm from the storage areas near the testicles to a place where they will have more access to human eggs. When coupled with erection during heterosexual intercourse, the sperm are deposited near the opening of the uterus, called the cervix, and are then able to find their way up the woman's tubes within minutes. If fertilization is to take place, it occurs while the egg is traveling down the tubes leading from the ovaries to the uterus.

Only a small fraction, roughly 5 percent, of the fluid discharged during ejaculation is composed of sperm. The majority is fluid from the seminal vesicles and prostate gland. Several small glands along the course of the urethra lubricate the pas-

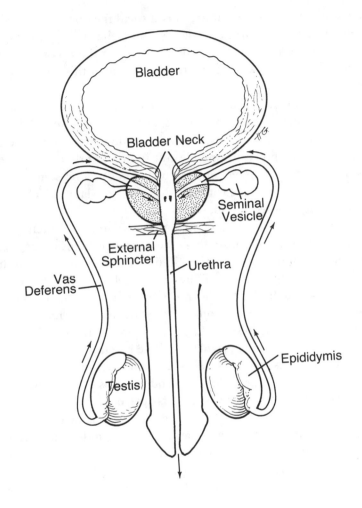

During ejaculation sperm made in the testicles travel from the epididymis and vas deferens to the urethra, where they mix with fluids produced by the prostate and seminal vesicles. The opening to the bladder closes, and the semen is forced out the tip of the penis by forceful muscular contractions.

sageway, but these contribute only a small fraction of the total as well. The fluid from these glands lining the urethra forms the small bead of milky fluid occasionally seen at the tip of the penis during sexual arousal. No sperm is present in this small collection.

The seminal vesicles are a pair of hollow glands approximately five centimeters in length that course away from the prostate like a pair of rabbit ears. Originally thought to store sperm, they are now known to provide nutrition and other factors necessary for sperm survival outside of the body. The seminal vesicles contribute the sugar fructose to the ejaculate, which is the main energy source for sperm.

The prostate is another major contributor to semen. Most men first hear of the prostate as they enter their fifties, as it can interfere with normal urinating. This occurs because the urethra runs through the center of the prostate like a doughnut hole through a doughnut. As the prostate grows, it can narrow the urethra so that voiding becomes more difficult. The reason for its location, however, is so that its juices can be deposited directly into the urethra during ejaculation. The prostate provides a number of chemicals that help the sperm on their journey.

Although its exact role in reproduction is still incompletely defined, prostate tissue was the first place within the body discovered to contain prostaglandins, hence their name (*prosta*, from *prostate*). Prostaglandins are chemicals that produce a variety of far-reaching effects throughout the body. Controlling prostaglandins has important medical consequences. For example, one of the ways that aspirin works is by interfering with prostaglandin production, although it now appears that the prostate is not a major producer of prostaglandins.

The seminal vesicles and prostate play out an interesting duet with semen. When a man ejaculates, the semen is initially thick like a gel. After ten to twenty minutes pass, however, the semen begins to liquefy. It turns out that the seminal vesicles produce a substance that causes the semen to gel, and the prostate provides the liquefying substance.

What is the significance of this? Well, in humans, probably not much. It seems reasonable that semen will stay within the vagina longer as a gel than as a thin liquid, although I suspect this has little effect on improving the chances for fertilization. In certain mammals, however, such as mice, there is a "copulatory plug" formed by the semen during intercourse that blocks the vagina physically and also has the effect of turning off the interest of other male mice.

What actually happens during ejaculation? As mentioned previously, the process is governed by the sympathetic nerves. At some point during genital stimulation, a threshold of excitement is reached within the nerves leading to the sexual center in the brain. Within the brain chemical fireworks are set off in an internal experience we call orgasm. At the same time, sympathetic nerves traveling to the testicles, vas deferens, epididymis, prostate, seminal vesicles, and urethra stimulate muscle fibers within these structures to produce a powerful discharge. In a coordinated fashion, sperm are transported within seconds from storage areas within the epididymis and vas deferens to be deposited within the urethra as it passes through the prostate. At the same time, the seminal vesicles and prostate contract, squeezing out their juices. These fluids mix in the prostatic urethra, and then suddenly they are expelled in rhythmic fashion along the urethra and out the penis.

The vas deferens is an interesting player in this process. This tube runs from testis to urethra and transports the sperm. It can be felt above the testicle in the scrotum as a firm structure, similar to a thick guitar string. It follows a circuitous route, passing through the inguinal canal up toward the hip, then diving deep into the pelvis behind the bladder, where it meets the prostate. Ninety percent of the thickness of the vas deferens is composed of muscle, with a tiny opening the size of a coarse hair through which the sperm travel. The muscle is necessary, of course, to get sperm from here to there within seconds. The sperm make a journey the equivalent of a marathon in two to five seconds.

Sometimes sperm make a wrong turn. Men with problems

affecting some branches of the sympathetic nerves can have the coordination of ejaculation mixed up. This can happen for a variety of reasons, but the most common are surgical procedures in the pelvis, where tiny nerves may be damaged inadvertently, and as the result of such diseases as diabetes.

Jerry was a thirty-two-year-old man who noticed that over the previous two years the amount of semen he ejaculated was progressively diminishing. Recently, he was only able to express a drop of semen, and often there would be nothing at all. The feeling of orgasm for Jerry was unchanged. He was diabetic and had been taking insulin for eight years. He was otherwise healthy and had never undergone any major operations. He did mention that when he urinated after sex, the water in the toilet bowl was more bubbly than usual, like a froth. This was a good sign, which I will explain shortly. His examination was completely normal.

I asked Jerry to come in on another day and to bring in a urine sample from home, taken immediately after intercourse. The urine was placed in a centrifuge, which makes all the heavier elements in the urine sink to the bottom by gravity. The top fluid was discarded, and a drop from the bottom portion of the centrifuged sample was placed on a slide. Under the microscope were hundreds of sperm. During ejaculation the sperm as well as the other fluids from the prostate and seminal vesicles were going backward into the bladder rather than out the tip of the penis. Why should this happen?

The urethra is a tube that is open at the tip of the penis and at the other end opens into the bladder. A muscle at the opening of the bladder, called the bladder neck or internal sphincter, normally closes during ejaculation so that the semen can only travel in a forward direction. The nerves that control this closure are also branches of the sympathetic nerves. If the bladder neck fails to close properly, the pressures generated in the urethra to propel the semen cause the semen to take the path of least resistance, which happens to be back into the bladder. This is called retrograde ejaculation. This causes no damage but can obviously be disconcerting and makes fertility problematic. The sperm are washed out with the next urination, so there is no accumulation of sperm where they do not belong.

Jerry provided a hint that this was his problem by volunteering the information that there were unusual bubbles in the toilet bowl when he urinated after sex. Protein can be stirred up into a froth, and semen contains a lot of protein. Egg whites are a good example of how proteins can be stirred up into a froth.

There is a wonderful story of a Chinese doctor coming as a visiting professor to a high-tech American medical center and making a diagnosis of kidney failure in a patient using nothing more than a wooden bowl filled with a sample of urine and an instrument similar to chopsticks. By rapidly stirring the urine the doctor produced a foam. One of the hallmarks of kidney failure is protein in the urine.

Jerry was interested in making babies and wanted treatment so that he could ejaculate in a normal fashion. Fortunately, some medications have actions similar to those of some of the sympathetic nerves, and thus they may help the bladder neck close. Jerry took a medication thirty minutes before intercourse and was able to have normal ejaculation again while the medication remained in his system.

Frank was not as fortunate. This twenty-eight-year-old man had had a testicular cancer removed, then had undergone radical surgery for removal of lymph nodes in the back of his abdomen. One of the side effects of this second operation is injury to the sympathetic nerves as they travel down the back portion of the abdomen, called the retroperitoneum (*retro* = behind; *peritoneum* = the sac containing the intestines and other abdominal organs). Frequently men who have had this operation will have retrograde ejaculation like Jerry, but others will have a greater disturbance of the ejaculatory mechanism, such that no semen is deposited within the urethra at all. Frank was now cured of his testicular cancer and wanted to have another child. He already had a five-year-old child from before the onset of his illness.

Frank's health was otherwise good. His abdomen had a large incision down the middle from his operation, and the left testis had been surgically removed. The remaining right testis, epididymis, and vas deferens felt normal. No sperm were seen in Frank's urine following ejaculation. He therefore did not have retrograde ejaculation. Instead, he had a condition called absent seminal emission. Sperm were not being deposited in the urethra at all. This occurred because the signal to deliver sperm, as well as the other components of semen into the urethra, was not getting to the proper destination. Although sensation in the penis during intercourse was normal for Frank, and although he experienced the same feelings of pleasure, sexual tension, and release during orgasm, the internal muscular response of some of the genital organs that normally occurs with orgasm was absent.

Frank tried the same medication as Jerry without success, then another as well. Urine was examined again to see if sperm were at least getting into the urethra but were ending up in the bladder. No luck. It was time for high technology.

Frank came to the operating room and had general anesthesia for approximately thirty minutes. A small probe was inserted into his rectum. Through this probe I transmitted electrical impulses directly in the areas where the nerves to the prostate, seminal vesicles, and vas deferens run. After approximately fifty impulses over five minutes, no fluid had discharged from the penis. A small, soft plastic tube called a catheter was passed through the urethra into the bladder and the urine collected. Some cloudy material floated in the test tube. From the laboratory came the message minutes later—sperm!

I had been able to obtain sperm from Frank, which could subsequently be used to inseminate his wife. Frank's medical story underscores the truly amazing process we take for granted all the time, namely the remarkable biological systems that normally work to allow the individual and the species to reproduce. For although perpetuation of the human species is not usually at the forefront of a man's thoughts during intercourse, this is the raison d'être for our entire reproductive system, including sexual arousal, erection, and ejaculation. What a remarkable piece of work.

CHAPTER 4

MICTURITION

■ *Micturition* is the fanciest medical word I know for urinating. Other words of less weight but with perhaps more meaning include *voiding, passing water, peeing, pissing, emptying one's bladder*, and *taking a leak*. Although strictly speaking this is not a function of the reproductive organs in man, it is intimately linked to several of the structures we have already met, including the prostate, urethra, sphincter, and bladder. As men age, the ability to get the urine out may assume greater importance than other activities involving the penis. In other words, for some men emptying the bladder adequately becomes much more important than sex.

Urine is simply waste filtered from blood. The kidneys, lying in the back just underneath the lowest ribs, receive one-quarter of the pumped blood from the heart and make urine from it. The red blood cells carrying oxygen, white blood cells that fight infection, protein, glucose, and many other critical components of blood pass out of the kidney essentially unchanged. On the other hand, waste products carried in the blood from muscles and other organs are filtered out and pass in the urine from kidney to bladder. The bladder then acts as a reservoir for urine, with no function other than to store it and, at the appropriate time, to squeeze it out through the urethra.

The bladder is composed of an inner lining called a mucosa, and surrounding muscle. The mucosa is similar to the mucosa of other parts of the body, such as the inner lining of the cheek. If irritated by infection, or scratched by a stone, it bleeds easily. The muscle is unusual in that it can expand to a tremendous degree, allowing considerable storage capacity while maintaining the ability to contract at various degrees of stretch. This allows us to void with only a small amount in the bladder, or with a large amount after a long car trip, for example.

When the bladder contracts, urine can pass out only if the sphincter muscles relax. We have already discussed the internal sphincter, or bladder neck, which was critical for ejaculation in a forward direction. Men also have a second sphincter, called the external sphincter, lying approximately three centimeters downstream from the bladder neck. The prostate lies between the two sphincters and plays no role in voiding until it becomes diseased or enlarges with age. Normal urination requires the coordination of a bladder contraction with simultaneous relaxation of the sphincter muscles.

Women are born with only one sphincter, which appears to be a combination of the two sphincters found in men. Why the difference? For one thing, the female urethra is considerably shorter than the male's, so physically there is not much room to set up two different control sites. Perhaps a better question is why do men need two sphincters? Is this like wearing a belt and suspenders at the same time?

The sphincters keep the urine inside. If they did not work, as soon as a drop of urine reached the bladder, it would drip onto our legs or clothing. Some people suffer from this problem, and it is no picnic. Their clothes smell, the constant moisture is uncomfortable, and yeast infections in the genital region are troublesome and difficult to eradicate due to the moisture. So perhaps it does make sense to be doubly sure of being dry by having two sphincters.

I suspect there must be more to it than this, however. Nature hates duplication. And if it were so important, then I would expect women to have the same physical arrangement as men. Further, following various types of surgery, one or the other sphincter may be disrupted, and it is very unusual for men to leak unless both sphincters have been damaged. In other words, one sphincter alone seems to do the job.

At a recent urologic meeting I raised the question of what was the purpose of two sphincters. Some heated debate raged, with three views espoused. First, this was an example of belt and suspenders, designed to be doubly sure that men did not suffer from incontinence. Second, the two sphincters acted as a special adaptation for urination. Support for this viewpoint came from the animal kingdom. Male lions have been observed to spray their urine in small squirts up to thirty feet away, marking out their territory much the way dogs do. The ability to do this is thought to come from intermittent trapping of urine between the two sphincters, generating high pressures by squeezing the surrounding muscles, and then quickly releasing the external sphincter. The problem with this argument is that humans do not spray (if they can help it), and intermittent flow in men indicates either obstruction or a weak bladder.

The third explanation, and the one I favor, is that the two sphincters serve as a sexual or reproductive adaptation in similar fashion to what was described above for urinating. Unlike the urinary stream, which normally is a smooth, continuous flow, ejaculation is a rhythmic, intermittent expulsion of fluid from the penis. A pressure-chamber effect should be more useful for ejaculation than urination since semen is so thick.

Assuming that the sphincters relax as they should, urination is then a balance between the expulsive forces of the bladder and the resistance of the outlet and the urethra. Normally, as with most younger men, the resistance is small, and the flow quite

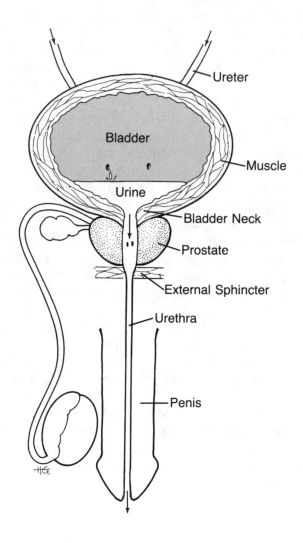

Ureter

Bladder

Muscle

Urine

Bladder Neck

Prostate

External Sphincter

Urethra

Penis

During urination the bladder muscle squeezes while the bladder neck and the external sphincter open up. The urethra runs through the center of the prostate before it joins the penis.

powerful. Young boys in particular are able to direct their stream many feet away. As the prostate grows with age, it reduces the caliber of the urethra, the resistance to flow is increased, and the stream is diminished as a result.

A number of factors determine how often a man urinates. Some of these have to do with the bladder, and some with the mind. Bob was a forty-two-year-old investment broker who came to see me because of frequent urination. He was very distraught and felt something terrible was going on with his bladder.

Every day for the last six months Bob had noticed that at the start of the trading day he had the urge to urinate two or three times each hour. This was very inconvenient, to say the least. When he made it to the toilet, usually only a small amount of urine came out. Almost as soon as he returned to his office, he felt the urge to urinate again. After the close of the trading session the urge to void would diminish, and he could then wait as long as three hours before urinating again. He slept through the night without awakening. Bob's examination was completely normal, including a normal-sized prostate, and his urinalysis was normal as well.

Bob's problem is quite common, although perhaps a little extreme. Everyone has the experience of needing to urinate frequently when anxious, for instance before an exam or a job interview. Usually only a few drops come out, since there has not been time for the bladder to fill. Although our sense of when it is time to void usually comes from a full bladder, this sensation can be influenced greatly by our state of mind.

Bob easily admitted to tension at work, particularly since his productivity had dropped over the last year. He had started to be concerned that his job might be in trouble. Bob's anxiety was manifested by his bladder irritability. In effect, his bladder became the focal point for his anxiety, just as under similar circumstances other people might develop headaches, abdominal pain, or diarrhea.

The treatment for Bob was primarily education and reassurance. After I explained how the bladder works and described what I felt was occurring to him, Bob brightened up, happy to know there was nothing terribly wrong. He asked what he should do when the strong urge to void interrupted his work. I suggested that instead of becoming more frustrated at the interruption in his work, he should stop, take several slow, deep breaths, and actively concentrate on relaxing his abdominal and pelvic muscles. The urge to void should pass, and Bob would be able to continue with his work.

I was not sure whether this would really work for Bob. Certain jobs do not easily allow incorporation of relaxation techniques. Motorcycle racing and high-wire circus performance come immediately to mind. There are also certain personality types, generally nervous individuals who turn their anxieties inward, who are prone to these sorts of problems, which can then be difficult to treat.

Bob called me several weeks later to say that his problem had resolved itself completely. The day after seeing me he had the usual urge to void shortly after the market opened. He closed his eyes, confident that the feeling would pass, and sure enough after no more than four or five seconds the urge to void left him. This happened several times during the course of the day. He was extremely grateful.

Two months later Bob returned to my office with a milder version of his original complaint. I reexamined him to make sure he had not developed a physical ailment such as an infection of the bladder or prostate, but everything checked out fine. We went through the same discussion we had had on his initial visit, and again Bob seemed relieved. Three weeks later Bob called to say that his symptoms were completely gone. Unfortunately, it was a bad time for the stock market. The resolution of Bob's symptoms coincided with his losing his job.

In the absence of significant anxiety, the usual determinant of how frequently a man voids is how often the bladder is filled. Most bladders have a "capacity" of two hundred to four hundred milliliters, or roughly seven to thirteen ounces. The amount is fairly constant for most individuals. When the bladder is filled to capacity, a man develops a strong urge to void.

The reason I highlight the word *capacity* is that the bladder can be stretched to a much greater volume under anesthesia, although a normally conscious person would not allow this to happen. If a person is unconscious from injury, anesthesia, alcohol, or any other reason, the bladder can be stretched to hold a liter of urine or more. The powerful urge to void when the bladder is full is really a protective measure for the bladder. Stretching the bladder beyond its normal limit can cause temporary or permanent injury.

Remember that the bladder is a muscle, and that muscles act by contracting, or shortening. Most of the larger muscles in the body are attached to bones or joints, and when they contract, they move an arm or leg or other part of the body in a given direction. The bladder muscle fibers are fixed not to bone but to each other. As the bladder becomes increasingly distended, the muscle fibers are drawn farther and farther apart, much as interlocking fingers have less and less contact with each other as the hands are pulled away. This results in a reduced ability to generate an adequate contraction, and voiding is thus impaired. Most bladders are unable to expel urine immediately after severe distension. Fortunately, after a period of rest in which the bladder is drained by a catheter, the bladder will usually return to its normal condition.

A demonstration of this phenomenon in milder form has been experienced by nearly every man. A car trip, meeting, or other situation has made it impossible for you to urinate even though your bladder is so full you are afraid you might wet your pants. You expect that as soon as you get to the toilet the urine will pour out like water from a fire hose. Instead, the urine comes out in a weak, dribbling stream, perhaps even in small, intermittent spurts. What happened? The bladder became overdistended and the muscle fibers were less effective than usual in generating a strong contraction.

Most people do not wait for the bladder to be completely full before voiding. You have probably noticed that sometimes you urinate a small amount, and at other times a much larger amount. Does this mean that the warning system of the bladder is randomly activated at different filling volumes? The answer is that there seem to be several stages of signals or warnings that vary in intensity from mild to moderate to severe. These signals take the form of a vague feeling that is often described as a pressure deep in the pelvis. The early signals are easy to dismiss, and the sensation passes within moments. As the bladder fills, the signals become more frequent and demanding. The brain appears to make a constant assessment about the relative merits of emptying the bladder and the convenience of doing so at that given moment. As the bladder fills, the equation tips increasingly toward voiding.

It is possible to test the sensation of the bladder by a test called a cystometrogram (CMG for short), which also measures the pressures within the bladder at different filling volumes. A CMG is usually performed for individuals with abnormalities of urination, although it is not absolutely necessary in many instances. During a CMG the bladder is slowly filled through a catheter with water or with carbon dioxide, a harmless gas. For the first fifty milliliters or so most people feel absolutely nothing. At some point after this, they feel a mild urge to void, but there is no discomfort. This first urge to void is called a first sensor. The urge disappears while the filling continues, and after the bladder has filled further, a stronger urge is noted, but this, too, can be ignored and passes. Finally the urge to void is great, and this is considered the capacity of the bladder.

Voiding can take place at any point as the bladder fills. Often when I ask a patient to leave me a urine sample and they say, "Oh, no, I just went to the toilet," they are able to produce a small sample anyway. Some people have what could be called an insistent first sensor. Like Bob, as soon as they have a small amount of urine in the bladder, they have the sensation that they must void, and the difficult part is that they are unable to ignore this urge. This is often a difficult problem for patient and physician, as it is unclear whether the problem is an overactive bladder sensor or that a normal signal is given too much credence by the brain.

As everyone knows, the voiding priorities of an infant are different from those of an adult. Otherwise we would all still be in diapers. The infant voids as a reflex every time he has the sensation of bladder fullness. Only as the baby develops some body awareness and control over himself is he able, with encouragement, to inhibit the natural reflex to empty the bladder at the first urge. This learned ability to inhibit the voiding reflex allows us to maintain control over when we void, and to free us from the need for protective undergarments. The reflex to void is controlled by a set of nerves that run from bladder to spinal cord and back to bladder. The mechanism to control or inhibit the reflex requires input from the brain, however. This inhibition center can be injured by a stroke, for example, resulting in what is termed urge incontinence. The stroke patient may simply void every time he has the urge, which may not be when he is standing in front of the toilet.

Certainly there are differences between individuals in regard to how much urine they can hold. People speak of big bladders and small bladders. The latter is often referred to as a "weak" bladder, although this is a misnomer, since the power of the bladder has nothing to do with its capacity. In medical school, as we learned dozens upon dozens of acronyms for various diseases, one of my classmates came up with the diagnosis of TWB (teeny weeny bladder) for a particular student who always left class early to go to the bathroom.

At the other end of the spectrum is the "truck driver's bladder." Truck drivers who were hired to haul cargo cross-country for a set fee would try to make the trip with as few stops as possible, since they could pick up another fare more quickly at the other end. Some would carry jugs in the cabin so they could void and drive at the same time (not a practice recommended in driver education classes), while others would try to hold off on voiding as long as they could. Some of these men trained themselves to void no more than twice daily and could void as much as a liter at a time.

Another determinant of how often one must empty the bladder is how much urine is being made and how quickly. The kidneys not only filter the blood to rid it of waste products, they also regulate the amount of fluid in the body. When the body is dehydrated from heat, sweating, or from a lack of fluids, the kidneys concentrate the urine by reclaiming much of the water. Less urine is made, but the chemicals deposited in the urine are excreted at approximately the same rate. This causes the urine to appear dark yellow. On the other hand, when the kidneys sense extra fluid on board from an increased intake of liquids, they excrete more urine. Under these conditions urine may even be colorless. So, the more you drink, the more you urinate.

There are certain foodstuffs and drugs that can affect how much urine the kidneys make, and these will then affect the frequency of urination. Foremost among these is alcohol. Alcohol acts as a diuretic, which means that it stimulates the kidneys to make more urine, even when the volume of blood in the body is well balanced. For this reason, people often feel thirsty after drinking moderate amounts of alcohol, since thirst is the body's way of telling us we are dehydrated. Diuretics are also a class of medications used specifically to reduce the amount of fluid in the body by increased excretion of urine by the kidneys. They are used for conditions such as hypertension and heart failure.

If you are taking a diuretic, you will urinate more often for several hours. Although bedtime is a convenient time of day to take many medications, the increased urine output from diuretics will force you to awaken more often at night to empty your bladder. Morning is therefore a more practical time to take this medication, although your physician should be your guide for this. Coffee, tea, and cocoa also seem to increase voiding frequency, possibly due to a small increase in urine output. These beverages should be avoided as much as possible if you urinate more often than you like.

CHAPTER 5

THE TESTICLES

■ If the penis is the psychic indicator of a man's maleness, then the testicles are the seat of his power. The phrase *he's got a lot of balls* is generally made with grudging respect to a man's boldness, gumption, or chutzpah. It is the source of his seed, of his reproductive capability. It is not for nothing that the testicles are often referred to as the "family jewels," since they represent the most valuable thing some feel a man can possess—his lineage. In one view characteristic of a strict biological interpretation for the nineties, the body is merely DNA's workhorse to produce more DNA. And the testicles are where the action is taking place.

Whatever their emotional significance, the testicles are a remarkable pair of organs with far-reaching effects throughout the body. They not only produce sperm, which carry the genetic information to the egg in order to create new life, but they also produce a number of hormones that travel through the bloodstream to reach distant points, affecting organs as diverse as the brain, muscles, and the vocal cords among others.

As discussed earlier, the testicles start out inside the body near the level of the kidneys and descend through the inguinal canal to take their place within the scrotum during the last months before birth. Occasionally they fail to make the trip on time and descend during the first year of life. In some cases parents and pediatricians may be concerned that the testicles have failed to descend properly, and it turns out that the testicles have made the trip just fine, thank you, but they are reluctant to let anyone know. As soon as someone looks at them cross-eyed, they pull up to safety in the inguinal canal, leaving the scrotum quite empty. How to distinguish between shy testicles and true undescended ones? If the testicle in question is ever down in the scrotum, then it is fine, and we call it a retractile testis. A wonderful pediatric urologist I know puts these boys in a tub of warm water. The testicles will often come down, and everyone goes home happy. However, approximately one out of a hundred boys will still have a truly undescended testis at one year, and something will need to be done to correct the situation.

The undescended testis becomes a liability. First of all, testicles quickly lose their ability to make sperm if not located in the scrotum. Second, the undescended testis is at increased risk of developing a cancer, although this risk of testis cancer is still extremely low. Finally, it has become clear that being "different" physically causes problems for children as they begin their social years by entering school. Not having two testicles qualifies as being different. There has thus been a push over recent years to bring the undescended testis down to its normal position as early in life as possible once it is clear that it will not descend spontaneously.

Testicles are induced to descend either medically or surgically. Medical therapy is occasionally successful, but surgery is usually required. In medical therapy a hormone called HCG is injected. This has some effects on the hormonal function of the testis. It is not at all clear why it works when it does, and in fact some doctors believe that it only "helps" in cases where the testis would have descended by itself. Others feel that it may be helpful in the mildest cases of cryptorchidism, where the testis has only a short distance to go in order to reach its proper location at the base of the scrotum.

In surgery for the majority of cases in which the testis has hung up in the inguinal canal, a small incision is made in the groin. For the more severe cases when the testis cannot be felt at all in the groin and is suspected to be located in the pelvis, an incision is made in the lower part of the abdomen. The goal is to free the testicle together with its blood supply and vas deferens so that it can reach the scrotum. If this works, the testis is then brought down to a small pouch under the skin of the scrotum and fixed in place. For testicles in the abdomen, there is often not enough length on the blood supply to bring them down directly. Choices are to remove the testis and replace it with an artificial testis, bring it down as far as possible and come back after a period of growth to try again, or transplant the testicle to the scrotum and make connections to new blood vessels with microsurgery.

If the testicle cannot be felt, it may mean that no testicle exists. Occasionally the blood vessels to the testis will twist on themselves and be squeezed shut. If this happens, the testicle shrivels up to a little nubbin. New techniques to look inside the abdomen with a telescope, called laparoscopy, can identify the blood vessels to the testis. If the blood vessels are identified and followed to a dead end, it means no testis is present, and nothing further needs to be done.

Once the testis gets to the scrotum it stays fairly quiet until puberty. However, a short burst of activity occurs earlier in development when the testis produces testosterone in order to imprint on certain organs the information that this growing person is indeed a boy. The most important organ to receive this information is the brain, which responds to the presence of testosterone by organizing certain brain centers in patterns that can later be recognized as male. It has been well demonstrated, for instance, that as a group, boys outperform girls on mathematical tasks, whereas girls do better than boys on verbal skills. Although these differences have been attributed in the past to environmental factors, e.g., girls may not be encouraged to excel in mathematics, there is growing evidence that these differences are due in part to hormonal differences. Other effects of the early, short-lived hormonal activation of the testis are to direct the genitalia to develop in a male pattern.

The testis is composed mainly of spaghettilike tubes with small openings that connect with each other near the back of the testis. The spaghetti ball is packaged tightly into an oval shape and is surrounded by a tough membrane. The spaghetti strands are called seminiferous tubules, and within these tiny tubes the sperm develop and finally travel out of the testis. Between the seminiferous tubules lie the testosterone-producing cells, called Leydig cells.

Sperm go through a complex series of steps to arrive at the final familiar appearance of a swimming cell with an oval head and a beating tail. Early on, they look quite different and have different names. These different cells are grouped together under the name "germ cells." *Germ cell* is an odd term, since most people think of germs as bacteria, viruses, "cooties," or other such unpleasant, infectious agents. In fact, *germ* refers to a small organism that may subsequently undergo further development (e.g., a germ of an idea), although unfortunately the term has been hijacked to refer in common parlance to bacteria and other pathological microorganisms.

During childhood there is little action within the seminiferous tubules. The germ cells are present only in their most primitive form, called spermatogonia. At this point they look nothing like the sperm one sees in high school biology, swimming freely propelled by a long tail. The spermatogonia are big, fat, round cells without a tail, fastened securely to the Sertoli cells, which will govern their further maturation. Only in the last stages of development do sperm have tails. And only after they have gone through complete maturation do the Sertoli cells cast them adrift, to swim through the lumen of the spaghetti strands and reach the way station of the epididymis on the way to the vas deferens.

The human body is composed of billions of cells, each a self-contained unit. The nucleus is the command center, with production departments where proteins are constructed, and a perimeter system called the cell membrane that allows only items with the appropriate passwords to enter or leave. Of the many types of specialized cells in the body, none has a story more interesting than sperm.

■ LIFE OF A SPERM

Red blood cells travel throughout the body carrying oxygen to muscles, brain, and other tissues, but they are quite passive, carried along by the pumping action of the heart. Liver cells make a huge array of proteins used to regulate the clotting system of the body and to detoxify chemicals in the blood, but these chemically active cells are rooted in place. Nerves are responsible for the complex brain waves that control our thoughts and actions, but individual nerve cells do little more than signal their neighbors whether the light is on or off.

Sperm, on the other hand, take an incredible journey and undergo a complete metamorphosis as they develop within the testis, travel to the epididymis where they mature further, and then are shot as from a cannon through the vas deferens, urethra, and out of the body. Their mission is not yet complete, as they must make their way past multiple obstacles to finally meet the ovum, where they undergo yet another chemical transformation, finally fusing membranes and allowing the tightly bound DNA to merge with that of the egg. Sperm are the only cells that are designed to function outside the body.

The life story of a sperm would make for an excellent adventure novel. There is everything required for a good read— romance, pathos, teamwork, daunting obstacles and external forces, success against tremendous odds. Finally there is a happy if philosophical ending when sperm meets egg. By merging, they lose their individual identities to form a greater, enduring whole. Are the handkerchiefs out yet? Now that I've given away the plot, let me fill in the details.

The story begins with the seminiferous tubules inside the testicle, where the sperm are "born." Two types of cells are found inside these tubules, the germ cells, which develop into sperm, and the Sertoli cells. The Sertoli cells are like strict schoolmasters controlling the development of the young germ cells. They surround and nurture the germ cells for the duration of their development within the testis. They also form a barrier protecting the germ cells from most chemicals in the blood, actively selecting only key substances to come into contact with the delicate immature sperm.

The most immature germ cells, called spermatogonia, are the only kind of germ cells within the testis until puberty. Once the testicles are stimulated during puberty by hormones from the brain, the spermatogonia begin to develop. It appears likely that we are born with all the spermatogonia we are ever going to have. To provide a continuing supply of sperm, the spermatogonia divide, creating new spermatogonia, which are then fated to go along the pathway to mature sperm. The original spermatogonia are responsible for maintaining the germ cell population. If for some reason, such as infection or radiation, the spermatogonia all die out, then no other cells will repopulate the seminiferous tubules to produce sperm, and the result is sterility.

As the germ cells develop from spermatogonia, they move centrally, so that the most fully developed germ cells (finally called sperm, or spermatozoa to be fancy) line the opening in the middle of the tubule with their tails hanging out. New cells destined to mature into sperm are constantly being made from the spermatogonia, and these displace the earlier round of germ cells up and eventually out. It is like moving up an elevator; once at the penthouse, it is time to step out into the party.

The spermatogonia are in contact with the chemicals and molecules floating outside the tubule. However, as the developing germ cells move up the elevator, the Sertoli cells wrap their arms around them and close off the free connection with the environment. From this point on, the germ cells will only be exposed to what the Sertoli cells allow through their tight junctions. These tight junctions produce what is called the blood-testis barrier.

Developing germ cells are highly sensitive to changes in their environment and are easily damaged. The blood-testis barrier protects the germ cells, particularly from any toxins that might pass quickly through the body before being removed by the kidneys or liver. Sperm are critical to reproduction, and reproduction is one of the most critical functions for any species. It makes sense, then, that arrangements would be made to protect sperm from passing dangers that might occur from eating the wrong berries, for instance, or drinking from an infected stagnant pool. In modern medicine, we use certain toxins to help individuals. Specifically, in cancer chemotherapy, drugs cause tremendous damage to certain tissues, more to the cancerous tissues than to healthy ones, we hope. The testis is often a "protected site" from chemotherapy, since these drugs are often unable to pass through the blood-testis barrier. A blood-brain barrier exists in similar fashion.

The blood-testis barrier also has a critical function with regard to the immune system. The immune system is the body's main defense force against invasion from such hostile agents as viruses, parasites, bacteria, and even cancers. When material is recognized as foreign and not belonging to the body, an immune response is provoked, involving antibodies and the white blood cells. To identify something as foreign, it is also necessary to be able to identify what is normal. This recognition of "self" is a complicated process, but it seems that there is a point early in life when the immune system says, for all intents and purposes, "Whatever is here now is self, and anything found to be different in the future will be considered foreign and will be attacked."

Consider what this means for the testis and the germ cells in particular. The more developed germ cells do not appear until puberty, and they undergo significant changes in their appearance and function. They are certainly different from any other cell in the body and were not present when the immune system was holding an amnesty period to recognize the different cells of the body. The blood-testis barrier created by the Sertoli cells protects the developing sperm from attack by the body's immune system, in effect shielding them from the vigilante militia of white blood cells.

In one of the most important changes sperm undergo as they develop, they lose half of the genetic information with which they started. This happens so that when the sperm and the egg fuse, and their DNA is combined, the new embryo will again have a normal amount of DNA. To make this change, germ cells undergo a splitting process called meiosis, in which the cell splits into two, with each new cell taking only one of each pair of DNA strands. These strands are called chromosomes. From an initial forty-six chromosomes consisting of twenty-three pairs, each germ cell ends up with twenty-three single chromosomes, none of which has a partner. The result is that each mature sperm contains only half the usual amount of genetic material present in other cells.

One of the interesting sidelights to this division of the DNA is that the sex chromosomes are also split up. The sex chromosomes, which make up one of the twenty-three pairs of chromosomes, contain the genetic code that confers maleness or femaleness to the resulting offspring. Females have two X chromosomes and are thus referred to as X,X, while males have a Y chromosome coupled with an X, so they are X,Y. All cells in a man, except the more mature germ cells, have a complement of chromosomes that are 46 X,Y. This means that spermatogonia are also 46 X,Y. As the pairs of chromosomes are split, half of the resulting germ cells will have an X chromosome, and the other half will have a Y chromosome. Whichever sperm reaches the egg will determine whether the offspring will be male or female. Sex determination of offspring is thus a male property.

How does this work? Remember that the female is X,X and that the egg must also undergo meiosis in which the forty-six chromosomes are split. In the female, every egg has an X chromosome. When sperm and egg combine their DNA, if the sperm contributes an X, the chromosomes will be 46 X,X, and the embryo is female. On the other hand, if a Y chromosome is added to the soup, the result is 46 X,Y, and a male is produced.

The fact that there are two types of mature sperm, namely "male" sperm and "female" sperm, has raised interest in the possibility of separating sperm with an eye toward directing the sex of offspring. Couples with two boys for instance might want to try for a third if they had a high likelihood of making a little girl. Some hereditary diseases are only carried by males or females, and sex selection would therefore also allow the birth of an unaffected individual.

In certain societies male offspring are more highly valued than girls because of their earning power, physical abilities in the field or as warriors, or for other reasons peculiar to that culture. Although these reasons may be objectionable, they have added to the push to identify ways to select sperm on the basis of sex. Veterinary researchers have also directed considerable effort at this project, since it may mean big bucks to farmers or animal breeders to be able to select either bulls or cows, roosters or egg-laying chickens, for instance, from existing livestock.

So far there has been only limited success in separating sperm. The idea, of course, is quite simple. If one could collect all the X "female" sperm in one test tube and all the Y "male" sperm in another, then it would be quite straightforward to take the appropriate test tube and place the sperm within the female reproductive tract to obtain the offspring of choice.

Techniques have been popularized to select the sex of your child based on disputed evidence that male sperm swim faster and are less hardy than female sperm. This resulted in recommendations that couples who desire male children should have sex close to the time of ovulation so that the quick male sperm get to the egg before the female sperm. If, on the other hand, a female is desired, one should have sex slightly earlier so the more fragile male sperm will fall by the wayside while the female sperm march up the fallopian tubes to await release of the egg from the ovary. In newer high-technology techniques, which are all still experimental, sperm pass single file through a special device called a cell sorter. Laser light is reflected differently by male and female sperm due to the small difference in the amount of DNA present, allowing the machine to sort the cells into one of two groups.

None of these techniques come close to being 100 percent effective, and at best they are able to achieve what is called enrichment of one sex or the other. Nevertheless, some individuals advertise that they can achieve greater than 80 percent success in selecting the sex of a human child, and they demand a hefty fee for this service. I suspect in ten to twenty years this may truly be possible. Until then, I would be very hesitant to pay anyone for such a service. Caveat emptor.

After division of the chromosomes occurs, the germ cells prepare for their fateful trip out of the body. Once ejaculated, they will no longer need any machinery to make new parts, and the control center can be tightly packaged since it will have almost no commands left to make. The sperm are released on autopilot. The nucleus shrinks down in size. The space between the nucleus and the cell wall also becomes much smaller. Gobs of material no longer needed by the spermatid are thrown overboard by the cell like so much ballast, to be recycled by the Sertoli cells for further waves of germ cells.

Now a tail begins to form, first as a small bulge, and later as a long extension of the cell. The remainder of the cell is now composed almost entirely of the condensed nucleus. Along the midsection connecting the tail to the head of the sperm is the energy machinery that will power the tail in its sweeping side-to-side motions when the time is right and fuel is available. Over the front portion of the oval sperm head is the equivalent of a warhead. This is the acrosome, and it is filled with enzymes designed to penetrate the defenses of the egg should they ever meet.

Once the nucleus is lean and streamlined, the tail fully

formed, and the midpiece ready for action, the fully developed germ cell is called a spermatozoon, or spermatozoa if there are more than one (and there usually are). The Sertoli cell holds the spermatozoa by the tips of its fingerlike projections, then casts them off into the tides of the testis. At this point the sperm look like sperm, but they do not act like sperm. Namely, they are still incapable of swimming. Swimming lessons are still to come.

The sperm travel to the back of the testis, then out of the testis to the epididymis. The epididymis lies outside the testis, on the back portion, attached near the top by the connecting tubes but also more firmly by fibrous tissue. When men examine their scrotum (and all men should perform a regular self-examination, but more on that later), they may feel this lumpy, soft mass adjacent to the testis. Often this causes alarm when a man first begins to examine himself, since a mass conjures up thoughts of cancer, but it is a normal part of male anatomy.

The epididymis is also composed of small tubules, not much larger than the seminiferous tubules, all packed in together like spaghetti again. However, only one long continuous tube makes up the epididymis, although it doubles back on itself thousands of times. If stretched out, it reaches twenty meters in length. In transit through the epididymis, sperm obtain the ability to swim, called motility.

If the epididymis is punctured at different points along its length and sperm withdrawn with an extremely fine needle, only those sperm that have traveled to the end of the epididymis will be swimming. Sperm in the midsection of the epididymis wave their tails in an ineffective manner, and sperm from the first part of the epididymis do not move at all.

After sperm pass through the epididymis, some may seep into the much larger tube of the vas deferens, affectionately referred to by urologists simply as the vas. Others jokingly call it the "vas deferens" between men and women. The vas is a thick muscular structure that is able to transport sperm rapidly from epididymis to urethra. As the sperm are forcefully ejected into the urethra, they are washed with an outpouring of fluid from the seminal vesicles and prostate during ejaculation. The first portion of the ejaculate has a high concentration of sperm, whereas the second half has less. This reflects the sequence in which the various glands and vas discharge their contents. Once ejaculated, sperm have only begun their journey. Much is yet to come.

■ INTO THE VOID: AN OUT-OF-BODY EXPERIENCE FOR SPERM

The sperm have been ejaculated and are now out of the body. Passive agents to this point, they will be passive no longer. If they have been deposited into the vagina, they must find their way into the opening of the uterus, called the cervix. The vaginal environment may not be all that pleasant for sperm. It tends to be acidic, and microorganisms may be present, such as yeast and bacteria, that are harmful to sperm.

The cervix may pose a formidable challenge. During most of the woman's menstrual cycle the cervix is filled with a thick mucus, obstructing the passage of sperm. They are repelled by it or end up being stuck, as in a giant pool of molasses. Around the time of ovulation, however, the mucus changes and becomes much thinner. Sperm swim in this mucus quite readily, and there is some evidence that sperm that find their way into the cervical mucus at this time serve as a sperm reservoir, so that if ovulation does not take place for another twenty-four hours, some sperm may still be in the female reproductive tract and can pass into the uterus and into the tubes.

Why should there be any cervical mucus at all during the fertile period for the woman? Part of the answer is that it acts as an effective filter, allowing sperm to enter around the time of ovulation while excluding many other substances within the vagina, such as bacteria or chemicals within the semen. Certain components of semen are counterproductive in the reproduction game within the uterus. Prostaglandins are one example. Their precise role is unknown, but their effect on the uterus is quite clear and problematic if they get inside together with sperm. Prostaglandins cause severe uterine contractions, which have the effect of expelling fluid.

Of those sperm that make it into the uterus, a portion make it quickly up the tubes to meet the egg if the timing is right. The egg is only within the tubes for approximately twenty-four hours. Once it passes through the tube into the uterus, there is essentially no further chance of fertilization, and the egg is expelled together with the lining of the uterus. Bleeding accompanies this, and we call this process menstruation.

For the lucky sperm that do encounter the egg at the appropriate time and place, their mission is neither easy nor complete. Many of the steps that follow are as yet poorly understood, but we do know parts of the story, which can truly be amazing. First, the sperm must penetrate the tough shell surrounding the egg. Remember that the sperm have a cap in front, like the front bumper of a car. This is the acrosome, and it is filled with enzymes. When sperm come upon the egg, they release their acrosomal enzymes, which dissolve small sections of the protective shell. This creates a hole large enough for sperm to swim through.

Once sperm and egg are in close approximation, they perform a secret handshake of recognition via chemicals on their surfaces. The membrane surrounding the sperm then merges with that of the egg. The DNA that has been tightly packed in the sperm head is released into the egg and immediately opens up. Under the microscope it appears that the sperm head is swelling. The tail of the sperm falls off. Remarkably, almost instantaneously with penetration of the sperm head there is a change in the membrane of the egg so that no further sperm are able to penetrate it. This protects against the confusing events that would follow from insertion of DNA from more than one sperm.

The sperm's mission is now complete. From an ejaculation of approximately 100 million sperm, one has made it through an assortment of obstacles to find its target. The remainder stay alive for up to forty-eight hours and are washed out from the system. From beginning of development to ejaculation took roughly two and a half months.

When the sperm's DNA merges with the egg's DNA, the resulting embryo has a full set of chromosomes and can begin dividing into two, then four, and then more cells. It passes into the uterus where, if circumstances are favorable, it settles into a soft bed of uterine lining and begins to make connections with blood vessels so that it can be nurtured over the next nine months. The ovaries stop releasing eggs. Sperm production continues unchanged. The man's biological role in fatherhood has been completed but his emotional one is about to begin.

■ VASECTOMY AND VASECTOMY REVERSAL

One cause of male infertility that is not a diagnostic puzzle is the fellow who walks into the office having had a vasectomy years ago. He is sterile thanks to his vasectomy and is interested in a vasectomy reversal. Alex was one example. He and his second wife, both schoolteachers, each had one child from their previous marriages but wanted to start a new family together. Alex had undergone an unsuccessful vasectomy reversal by his urologist and now wanted to try again. Before I tell you a little more about Alex, I would like to discuss vasectomy itself in greater detail.

Vasectomy comes from *vas,* referring to the vas deferens, and *-ectomy,* which means "removal of." Similarly, an appendectomy refers to removal of the appendix. Vasectomy, then, really means removal of the vas deferens. No one actually removes the entire vas, although many urologists will remove a portion of it. The goal is to obstruct the vas so that sperm can no longer travel to the urethra, and the man is rendered sterile.

The vas can be felt above each testis in the scrotum as a thick wire, like a guitar string. The urologist grasps the vas beneath the skin, injects a local anesthetic, and cuts the vas. The ends are tied with sutures or closed with tiny metal clips. The openings are often cauterized to be extra sure that sperm cannot leak out from one

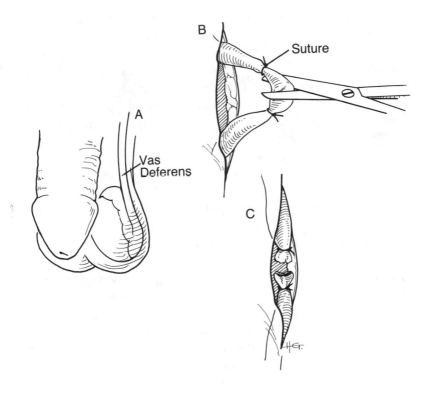

B

Suture

A

Vas
Deferens

C

Vasectomy is performed by tying closed the vas deferens and then cutting it. This must be performed on both sides of the scrotum.

end or climb back in from the other. The entire procedure takes twenty to thirty minutes, after which I instruct my patients to take it easy for two to three days to avoid any excessive swelling or bleeding. There is usually only minor discomfort afterward.

Several million vasectomies are performed worldwide each year because it is a safe, effective means of birth control. There have been some health scares in the past regarding vasectomy, but none appear to be well founded. In the 1970s researchers performed vasectomies on monkeys and found that they developed heart disease more quickly than monkeys that had not had vasectomies. Naturally, this caused tremendous concern, since we are closer to monkeys biologically than almost any other animal. Could millions of Americans be at risk for premature heart disease because of their vasectomies? Considerable research on vasectomy in numerous other animal species, as well as other strains of monkeys, finally dispelled that concern. More recently there has been some concern that vasectomy may predispose one to prostate cancer, but there is very little to suggest that this is true.

So it seems that vasectomy is safe. Is it guaranteed? Anyone who has ever had any dealings with the medical profession knows that nothing is guaranteed. However, vasectomy is as good as any other form of birth control available, and certainly less difficult than a tubal ligation in a woman. It is not a perfect procedure because of what is called recanalization, in which a new "canal" or passageway is made by the sperm leading from one end of the cut vas to the other. This is quite uncommon, but it is something to be aware of if a man is considering vasectomy.

It generally takes several weeks and many ejaculations to flush out the last sperm lying in the vas beyond where the tube was tied. Since those sperm are capable of fertilization, I have all my patients provide a semen sample at two months to be sure that no sperm are still present. Until then couples must continue to use some other form of birth control if they do not wish to risk a pregnancy.

What happens to sperm after vasectomy? The sperm eventually die and are recycled by the body's scavenger system. Surprisingly, for most men there is no noticeable change in the amount of semen ejaculated after vasectomy, since only the sperm have been blocked, and they comprise no more than 5 percent of the ejaculate volume. The sensation of ejaculation is unchanged as well. There is no pain associated with sex or ejaculation after vasectomy.

Since reversal of a vasectomy is a much more difficult procedure, and since success is far from assured, I caution men thinking of a vasectomy that they should consider it a permanent decision. Given the availability of other effective and reversible forms of birth control, a vasectomy should be considered only by men who are confident that they are not likely to be starting a new family at any time in the future.

Back to Alex. After making an incision on each side of Alex's scrotum I was able to examine each testicle, epididymis, and vas in turn. On both sides there was a knot of tissue at the end of the vas, then a gap where the vas was no longer present. It seemed that the previous reversal attempt had pulled apart. I cut back to fresh tissue at both ends of the vas and found sperm in the fluid coming from the testicle side. With the operating microscope I placed several fine sutures almost too small to see with the naked eye between the inner openings of the two ends of the vas until this was closed. Then I took slightly less fine suture material and brought together the muscle of the vas so that the connection would be both watertight and strong. After completing both sides, I replaced the testicles in the scrotum and sutured the skin.

At his postoperative visit, there were many sperm swimming in Alex's ejaculate. A year and a half later I received a family-photo Christmas card with a four-month-old boy sitting in Santa's lap and the words *Thank you* written on the top. Those cards are the best thanks possible.

Vasectomy reversal is easier than hooking up the vas to an obstructed epididymis, but it still requires excellent operating skill under the microscope. Even today some urologists erroneously believe it is adequate to simply put both ends of the vas together with some heavy-duty suture and hope for the best.

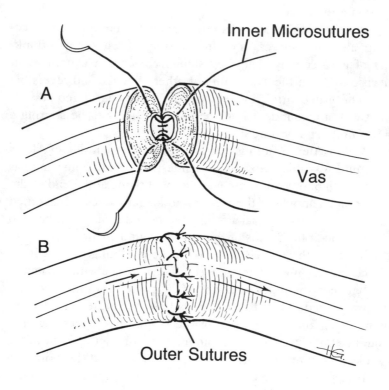

Inner Microsutures

A

Vas

B

Outer Sutures

Vasectomy reversal as it appears highly magnified under the microscope. The inner tube is closed first, followed by a second layer of sutures to make the connection watertight.

Reading through the operative notes from Alex's first vasectomy reversal attempt, I saw the surgeon took no longer than half an hour to do the entire procedure. To do the job properly under the microscope takes roughly three hours, sometimes longer. The time-consuming part is connecting the inner openings under the microscope with those fine sutures. If that part is not done properly, then the opening will be obstructed, or sperm will leak out and cause scarring.

Microsurgery has greatly improved the success of modern vasectomy reversal, but the surgeon has little control over some things. Probably the most important factor in predicting success for an experienced microsurgeon is the length of time since the original vasectomy. Some detrimental process appears to occur to the testis over time with obstruction. The longer it has been since vasectomy, the lower the chances of achieving a pregnancy with reversal.

Obviously, no man who undergoes a vasectomy has plans to reverse it within the foreseeable future. The average man I see for vasectomy reversal had his vasectomy performed eight to ten years previously. Success rates for these men are approximately 80 percent in terms of finding sperm in the ejaculate, and 50 percent pregnancy rates. For men beyond ten years the numbers drop to about 50 percent for the presence of sperm, and 20 to 30 percent for pregnancy rates.

The biggest obstacle for most men or couples considering this procedure is cost. Few insurance companies will pay for this, arguing that they never pushed for the vasectomy in the first place, and the reversal is not performed for treatment of illness. The cost of any procedure performed in the operating room has become ridiculous, and one should be prepared to pay in the range of $7,000 to $10,000, which covers the operating room charges, anesthesia fees, and surgeon's fees. Is it worth it? There is no right answer. Probably the most personal decision in the world is whether or not to have children, and who can say whether something is worthwhile? Certainly the risks of the procedure are minor, and there is usually little discomfort afterward.

PART II

Problems

CHAPTER 1

SEXUALLY TRANSMITTED DISEASES

■ There is good news and bad news about sexually transmitted diseases (now the preferred term for what had previously been called venereal diseases). The good news is that antibiotic therapy can cure all the classic illnesses that had caused so much suffering and even death in the pre-antibiotic era. The bad news, of course, is that a new sexually transmitted illness has appeared on the scene for which we so far have only a limited ability to treat—AIDS. AIDS stands for acquired immunodeficiency syndrome and is now recognized to be caused by a virus called human immunodeficiency virus, or HIV. AIDS has again ushered in an era where sexual contact brings with it the potential for illness and death. Needless to say, many men and women now experience considerable anxiety about having sex.

Alfred was a thirty-year-old single businessman whose life turned sour after a business trip to Thailand. He had intercourse there with a prostitute without using a condom, and upon returning to the United States several days later, he became concerned that he might have contracted some awful sexual disease, or even AIDS. He developed terrible headaches, pain in the back of his neck, was no longer able to achieve an erection, and had lost all interest in sex.

Alfred went to his internist, who performed a battery of tests, including those for AIDS, hepatitis, and syphilis. Everything came back negative. Somewhat reassured that his life was not immediately endangered, he was still left with a lack of sexual desire, which he found unusual and disturbing. He no longer awakened with erections and found it difficult to achieve an erection with masturbation. He also felt that the sensation in his penis had changed, sometimes having the feeling of pins and needles, and at other times feeling completely numb.

I was the third doctor Alfred had seen for this problem. Both of the previous doctors had been unable to find a physical problem. Alfred refused to believe there was nothing wrong with him physically, since he had so many clear-cut physical symptoms. Nevertheless, his physical exam was completely normal. It was clear to me that Alfred had experienced the scare of his life by having unprotected sex with a prostitute, and it made perfect sense that this fear might surface as abnormal feelings in and around the sexual organs.

For most mammals, sexual desire is greatly diminished under conditions of stress, hunger, fatigue, or fear. In a Darwinian sense, this is perfectly logical, since an animal should not be expending significant energies toward reproduction when other survival issues are at hand. What Alfred needed was reassurance, reassurance that he was going to be all right, that there was no evidence for any particular illness, that he would be able to be a sexual person again in the future, that his symptoms would resolve over time.

I spoke with Alfred several weeks after our first meeting. His erections had returned, and his headaches had disappeared, but there were still some odd sensations in his penis. He was still convinced he had some illness that had so far avoided detection, and he was eager to have more testing done. However, I did not think there were any tests that would have addressed his basic concerns.

I am not sure if I helped Alfred all that much. He went on to see at least two other doctors that I know of, as well as a therapist, and he may still feel that he is not yet whole. Nevertheless, Alfred's symptoms were clearly psychosomatic, caused by his fear of sexually transmitted disease, and fueled by his ignorance of what those diseases actually are. Although Alfred's symptoms were severe, many men and women share Alfred's concerns about becoming seriously ill from engaging in sex. Having some knowledge about sexually transmitted diseases can be helpful by putting this fear into a more reasonable perspective.

■ GONORRHEA AND SYPHILIS

When most men think of a sexually transmitted disease, they think of gonorrhea, often referred to as "the clap." Gonorrhea is caused by the gonococcus bacteria, which has a special attraction for the urethra. The body tries to fight this bacteria with white blood cells, which are part of the immune system. The collection of white blood cells appears as a creamy discharge from the urethra, and this is the hallmark of gonorrhea. The discharge usually appears within one week of contact with an infected partner. It is generally easily treated with penicillin or other antibiotics and, if treated early, will not usually cause any further problems.

Untreated gonorrhea may spread to form a rash or may infect the joints or even the lining of the spinal column causing meningitis. Within the genital system, it may cause infection of the testicles and the epididymis, as well as scarring of the urethra. These effects may result in infertility or difficulty with voiding. Gonorrhea in women is more difficult to detect and, if untreated, may result in scarring of the tubes, leading to infection of the pelvic organs or infertility.

The other major cause of urethral discharge is an organism

called chlamydia. Chlamydia provokes a less intense response from the body, so the discharge tends to be watery. Chlamydia is fussier than gonorrhea in terms of what it needs to grow in the laboratory, so that culturing the organism in a dish for identification has been more difficult. As a result, in the past when a patient had a discharge and gonorrhea could not be identified, it was called a "nonspecific" urethritis. Nowadays, cultures for chlamydia are routine, and the term *nonspecific urethritis* has been largely abandoned.

Syphilis is often confused with gonorrhea, although the two diseases have little in common apart from primarily infecting the genital organs and being sexually transmitted. Whereas gonorrhea causes a urethral discharge, syphilis usually presents as an ulcer or crater on the penis. The ulcer is called a chancre (pronounced shanker). It is beefy red, with firm edges, and looks quite painful. Surprisingly, it is not usually painful, and for this reason the chancre is occasionally ignored until it disappears. However, instead of this being the end of the story for the relieved individual, it is often the beginning of a more insidious process with potentially drastic consequences.

Once the chancre disappears, the responsible bacteria, called a spirochete (spy-ro-keet) because of its spiral shape, may be gone for good or may simply have gone "underground," only to reappear at distant sites weeks to months later. Usually, the result is a rash, prominent on the palms of the hand and soles of the feet. Alternatively, there may be some raised areas, particularly in the groin or around the scrotum and anus, which are teeming with spirochetes. This stage may also resolve without treatment, and all may appear quiet again for more months or years until there may be destruction of bones, dementia, and even damage to the back part of the spinal column where the nerves carrying information about sensation travel to the brain. This results in impaired sensation of organs such as the bladder, and these affected individuals may develop hugely distended, poorly functional bladders because they are unaware that it has become overfilled.

■ HERPES

Herpes is caused by a virus that afflicts the genital areas of men and women, and it can be transmitted by oral or genital intercourse. It produces one or several clear blisters that eventually burst, leaving a small, shallow red crater. These blisters are often painful or itchy. It can take one to two weeks for the blisters and craters to clear up, but they do disappear without treatment.

One of the most disturbing aspects of a herpes infection is that the virus takes up residence in the nerves and may sit there quietly for months or even years before returning in the same general area. This means that once you have herpes, you have it for life. Some people are unfortunate enough to have recurrences every month or two, although in most cases this slows down. There is no cure for herpes, but medications in the form of creams or pills may shorten the time that the sores are present.

The important thing to remember is to avoid sex while having a herpes outbreak so that you do not infect your partner. Condoms may be protective, but abstinence until the sores are completely gone makes better sense. If frequent recurrences are a problem for you, you should see a dermatologist or urologist about medical treatment.

■ AIDS

AIDS is one of the most amazing medical stories of the century. It appears to be a brand-new disease for humans that has arisen only within the last twenty years. Out of the blue, this disease has become a leading cause of death for adult men and women under fifty years of age. Although it is critical that further intensive research be directed at this disease, it is still remarkable how much we have learned in such a short time.

In 1982 I was a surgical intern at a major teaching hospital in Boston, and AIDS was only beginning to be a serious health problem. At that point the most commonly afflicted individuals were gay men and intravenous drug users. No one knew what caused the disease, and so it was unclear exactly how it was transmitted. Ignorance causes fear, and there was plenty of fear to go around.

A researcher at my hospital was looking for ways to identify men with AIDS, since there was no blood test at the time. All that was known was that individuals with AIDS developed lethal infections from organisms that would normally be easily handled by the body's immune system. This is where the name AIDS comes from—*a*cquired *i*mmuno*d*eficiency *s*yndrome. We therefore did biopsies of lymph nodes from men suspected of having AIDS, and these lymph nodes were then used for research purposes. The atmosphere in the operating room was always incredibly tense for what should have been a minor procedure. Many nurses refused to take part. Everyone wore extra pairs of gloves, and the handling of the removed tissues was carried out as if they were highly radioactive.

A short while later it was discovered that AIDS is caused by a virus, called the human immunodeficiency virus, or HIV. We learned that this virus is present in many body fluids, such as semen and blood, and therefore it became easier to understand that sex or using contaminated intravenous needles could transmit the disease from one person to another. The HIV virus can be passed on with either homosexual or heterosexual intercourse. However, if there is no sharing of body fluids, then there is no way to transmit the virus. You cannot get the virus by hugging, shaking hands, or by sharing the same toilet.

This helps explain preventive measures against AIDS and other sexually transmitted diseases. If you can protect yourself from coming into direct contact with body fluids containing the infectious organism, then you will prevent the bacteria or virus from making your body its home. A key component of this is using a condom when having intercourse. This prevents the semen from coming into contact with the vagina, or with the rectum during anal intercourse. Also the covered penis is not exposed to secretions from a partner. Clearly, the condom must be without holes to be effective, so it is recommended that you use a new condom with each sexual event, and to replace even a new one immediately if a hole in it is discovered. Since mistakes do happen, the term *safe sex* referring to the use of a condom should more properly be called *safer sex*. Another good idea is to wash your penis with soap and water following intercourse.

AIDS has no specific symptoms, and there is usually a delay of many years before HIV has impaired the immune system enough for an affected person to become ill. Even today, the most common way that individuals discover they have AIDS is if they come down with an unusual infection. The diagnosis of HIV infection can now be made by a simple blood test. Although there is still no cure for AIDS, research is progressing rapidly, and everyone hopes it will not be too long before a vaccine or effective treatment is available. In the meantime, prevention is the best treatment.

CHAPTER 2

INFERTILITY

■ Many cultures, including our own, believe for the most part that infertility is a woman's problem. The reasons for this are several, including patriarchal value systems, the obvious relationship between pregnancy and women, and the feeling that baby-making is simply women's work. Let me also add ignorance. The fact of the matter is that in 40 percent of infertile couples there exists a male problem without any known female factor. In another 40 to 50 percent there is an isolated female problem, and in another 10 to 20 percent there is what is called combined subfertility, where both partners may have some abnormality contributing to infertility. Considering that 15 percent of couples are infertile, this translates into a lot of men with fertility problems.

Infertility is not really a disease since it causes no symptoms, but it is certainly a medical problem. Classically, a couple was not considered infertile until they had been trying unsuccessfully for a full year. Nowadays, most couples and their doctors would begin looking into the problem well before a year of concerted effort has gone by.

Because infertility applies to couples rather than individuals, it is more difficult by a factor of two to identify a cause. Since the only symptom is the absence of a desired event, namely a baby, there may be few clues to lead physicians where to look. And not infrequently, no specific problem or abnormality is identified, which can be extremely frustrating for both the couple and their doctor.

There are several reasons for this. First is that conceiving a child is a probability game. Although millions of sperm are normally deposited within the vagina to meet the single egg at the appropriate place and time, any number of things may go wrong. The proof that the process is far from a sure thing is that we produce so many sperm. If fertilization were easy, men could get by with ejaculating only a dozen or so sperm at a time, instead of 100 million. Evolution has dealt with the problem of long odds against any single sperm-egg combination by flooding the system. The chances of winning the lottery improve dramatically if you buy thousands of tickets. Even with all those sperm swimming around like some giant (or microscopic) search party for the egg, the average fertile couple takes three to six menstrual cycles to conceive.

Let's look at where the problems may occur for a man. First, production of sperm within the testis has to be normal. Next, the sperm must be transported out of the testis into the epididymis, which acts as a reservoir. The storage and maturation of the sperm must be adequate, or the sperm will "spoil." The sperm must then be deposited into the urethra during ejaculation. The bladder neck must close during ejaculation so that sperm will not travel backward into the bladder. The sperm mix with secretions produced by the prostate and seminal vesicles for a proper ejaculate to be formed. Once deposited within the vagina, they must swim into the cervical mucus, then into the uterus and up the fallopian tubes to meet the egg. The sperm must recognize the egg, attach themselves, and penetrate its covering. Sperm and egg fuse, and an embryo is formed. The embryo must then find its way into the uterus and attach itself to the lining of the uterus wall. Only now has a pregnancy occurred. It is a complicated process, and things can go wrong at many points.

Richard's story provides a good example of some of the issues with male infertility. Richard and his wife had been trying without success to make a baby for nearly a year. A semen analysis showed absolutely no sperm was present in Richard's ejaculate. He had always been healthy, took no medications, had never had any injuries or infections related to his genitals. A repeat semen analysis gave the same result. He was in shock. What was wrong with him? It would have been easier to understand if he had been in some accident or had developed some illness.

Richard's condition of having absolutely no sperm in the ejaculate is called azoospermia and can sometimes be a "good" thing. No sperm at all may mean that the testicles are doing a really poor job of making sperm, or it may mean the sperm are simply not getting out, perhaps due to a blockage that could be corrected. What was promising for Richard was that his testicles were normal in size and firmness. If testicles are functioning poorly, they are often small and soft. Richard's only abnormality was that the tube that transports the sperm from the testicles, the vas deferens, could not be felt on one side. The other side felt completely normal.

The first test was to make sure that the sperm were not simply traveling backward into the bladder during ejaculation. Richard was instructed to bring into the office a urine sample after having sex. This was centrifuged, so that all "heavy" things such as sperm would end up at the bottom to be examined more easily. No sperm were present. The next question was whether sperm production or sperm transport was a problem. Richard underwent a biopsy of the testis, in which a tiny sliver of the inner testis was removed to be examined under a microscope. This is generally done under general anesthesia and takes no more than twenty to thirty minutes. Although few men look forward to a testis biopsy, it is a minor procedure, after which the man goes home with a jockstrap and a soreness that lasts several days. Most men go back to work the next day, or the day after that.

Richard underwent a close examination of his testicles and the connecting structures while under anesthesia for the biopsy. The left testis and tubes looked fine, but the right side was abnormal. The epididymis simply ended after only one-third of its normal length, and there was no vas deferens at all. Clearly, any sperm made from the right side had nowhere to go. But there must also have been a problem on the left, otherwise there should be reasonable numbers of sperm appearing in the ejaculate.

The biopsies showed that both testicles were producing sperm in a normal fashion. The right side had an obvious delivery problem, but how to evaluate and treat the left side? Richard had a special type of X ray performed under anesthesia, called a vasogram. A needle is inserted into a small opening made in the vas deferens, and dye is injected. If the tube is open, then dye will be seen along the length of the tube and also in the urethra and bladder. Richard's vasogram showed that his left tube was open. If no sperm were coming out despite the tube's being open, then there had to be a blockage closer to the testis. The epididymis is the most common place for such a blockage to occur, since it is so delicate, and therefore vulnerable to scarring from even minor infections. Indeed, on close inspection, a dis-colored area in the left epididymis suggested scarred tubules. Richard needed an operation to bypass this scarred area and make a new connection from the good part of the epididymis to the vas deferens.

Under the microscope a segment of the epididymis was iden-tified that looked healthy and had swollen tubules, indicating that they might be full of sperm. A single tubule was marked with an incredibly small suture and then opened. The escaping fluid was examined under a regular laboratory microscope, and I was pleased to see many swimming sperm. This was clearly a good tubule to connect to the vas deferens.

The vas deferens was cut close to the epididymis, and the cut end was brought past the discolored, scarred area to the marked tubule with seeping sperm. Several sutures were placed with the aid of the operating microscope to connect the tubule and the vas. The sutures were then tied down extremely carefully so that they would not tear or break. A second layer of slightly heavier suture was then placed to reinforce the new connection and make it watertight. After the four-hour operation Richard went home. I saw him back in the office three weeks later. He had healed up nicely, and there were now sperm in his ejaculate. The operation was a success, and Richard and his wife went on to have a little boy.

Not everyone has a happy ending. Richard had a physical blockage, and often these kinds of problems can be fixed with a mechanical solution, such as surgery. Many times it is difficult to find the exact cause of poor sperm quality, or surgery may not work out. Sometimes a man must face a long road of tests and procedures. Each man responds differently to the prospects of a given test or procedure, and it is neither possible nor reasonable for a physician to tell someone in this situation what is the right thing for him to do. Some men may choose to go ahead with a procedure with a low chance of success, and others may turn down a procedure that is more promising.

When I first met David, he had undergone many months of tests and procedures in another state, yet he was determined to pursue his problem to the end even though he knew it might mean more surgery. At each point along the way David understood that his chances for success were slim, yet he maintained an upbeat attitude. When the last procedure failed, and I called David to inform him of his semen analysis results, he sounded relieved rather than upset. He provided me with a brief analysis of his emotional journey. "I had to do what I could," he said. "I feel good knowing that I followed it out to the end."

There is often a terrible sadness when an individual discovers that he or she is infertile. The change in one's self-image must be addressed, the loss of hopes and dreams that had existed since childhood of what it would be like to be a parent. And there is also the feeling of a loss of control about one's body, as occurs with any medical problem. This loss is heightened, however, among young healthy men in their reproductive years, who have often never been disappointed by their body. Some men are shattered by infertility, and I frequently recommend counseling for men, alone or with their partners, to deal with this blow.

David's response was rather adaptive, I believe, in that he sought to do all that he could within reason and would then live with the results. It is a difficult thing to do, and very impressive. I do my best to educate my patients as well as treat them, but more often than not I discover that it is my patients who teach me.

Emotionally speaking, David was fortunate in that there was a definite end to his possibilities. More often than not, the problems of infertile couples reduce their chances of achieving a pregnancy in a reasonable time but do not exclude that possibility. Each ovulatory cycle then becomes the focus of hope, fear, and anxiety. Intercourse becomes a calculated event, timed to coincide with the most fertile day or so for the woman, i.e., when she ovulates. Sex becomes a chore rather than a pleasure and carries with it the reminder that the couple may be reproductive failures. It is not uncommon for men to become impotent while all this is going on.

For many, a happy event results. For others, especially men with drastically reduced sperm counts, fertilization becomes highly unlikely, and yet there is no one to say when enough is enough. The tease of "it's unlikely but possible" drags on and can interfere with normal daily activities for many months, and sometimes years.

Despite all this, there is much that can be done for the infertile couple, and the infertile man in particular. In the pages that follow I will describe some of the problems, the evaluation of the infertile man, and some of the currently available treatments as well as new developments on the horizon. Although my emphasis here is on men and their fertility problems, it is important to keep sight of the fact that the woman and her fertility are also crucial to the outcome. It should therefore be understood that even when there is an obvious problem with the man, his partner must also undergo careful evaluation.

■ DIAGNOSIS OF MALE INFERTILITY

When a couple has tried unsuccessfully to get pregnant for a period of time, the woman will usually go see her gynecologist or family doctor. The doctor will ask a few questions to determine whether there are any obvious problems that might interfere with becoming pregnant and will then perform a physical examination. Often the woman will need to keep a chart of her morning temperatures to see if and when she ovulates, and she might need blood tests or X rays as well, to see if there might be hormonal problems or blockages of the tubes. At some point early in this investigation the man should be asked to do a simple test called a semen analysis.

The semen analysis is the basic test to evaluate a man's fertility. The man ejaculates into a cup by masturbation or by interrupting sex, and the specimen is then examined in the laboratory. The ejaculate starts off as a gel, but then liquefies over the next ten to twenty minutes. It then is analyzed for the volume, pH, concentration of sperm, percentage of sperm that are swimming (motility), and percentage of sperm that have a normal appearance (morphology). For reasons that are not clear, human semen always includes significant numbers of sperm that look abnormal and do not swim. Obviously, if there are few normal, swimming sperm available, it will be more difficult to get pregnant.

The semen analysis may indicate several problems. There may be a low volume of the ejaculate, indicating an incomplete collection, obstruction of the ejaculatory ducts, or that the semen is being ejaculated back into the bladder. The number of sperm may be low, the motility may be low, the morphology may be low, or there may be some combination of these. Alternatively, the semen analysis may be completely normal, in which case it is unlikely that a male problem is present. Since there is often a large variation in the results of the semen analysis, it is often necessary to obtain two or three samples before determining what the true numbers are. A male fertility problem is diagnosed when some abnormality in the semen analysis is repeatedly present.

Certain religions prohibit sexual activity that is not performed for purposes of reproduction, such as masturbation or intercourse with a condom. In these cases an incomplete collection of semen can be obtained by having sex with a perforated condom with the blessing of one's religious leader. An incomplete sample can still provide useful information on the quality and concentration of sperm, and the religious prohibition is satisfied since the possibility of a pregnancy from the sexual activity is still present.

Since most women of reproductive age have a gynecologist, and relatively few men of that age have a doctor of any type, couples with infertility usually begin their evaluation with the gynecologist. Most of the men I see have therefore already had a problem identified by semen analysis. The goal is then to find out what has caused the problem and what can be done about it.

In the office I ask men about their general health as well as their reproductive history. If you have fathered children in the past but are now having difficulty, this puts you in a completely different category from a man who has never fathered one. A different set of problems might make a man newly infertile. I ask whether the couple is having sex at the appropriate time in the menstrual cycle, and how often they have intercourse. I obtain a list of the man's medications and previous operations. I also need to know if a man is using recreational drugs such as marijuana, cocaine, or anabolic steroids, all of which may affect sperm function or production.

A history of infections with high fevers may cause temporary or permanent injury to the testis. Mumps is a fairly benign disease of childhood, but if it occurs after puberty, it can cause infection in the testicles, which frequently results in sterility.

Surgery of the lower abdomen, hernia repairs, or urologic procedures, particularly of the genitals, may all cause problems with
fertility under certain circumstances. Developmental history is
important, such as whether both testicles were descended at
birth and whether puberty was delayed.

The examination focuses on the genitals. In particular, I assess the size and consistency of the testicles and evaluate the
epididymis and vas deferens on each side. I usually examine men
both while they are standing and lying down to help identify the
presence of a varicose vein in the scrotum, called a varicocele,
which may be important. I do a rectal exam to check the prostate
and examine the urine microscopically for the presence of bacteria and white or red blood cells, any of which may suggest a
problem. By the time the history and physical examination have
been done, I often have a good idea of what the problem might
be. Nevertheless, a series of tests must often be performed to
clarify the issues and also to determine what the likelihood of
success may be for a given individual.

Special tests on sperm may be necessary to see how well they
function. These tests may include placing the sperm in mucus to
assess the ability to move through the mucus at the opening of
the uterus. Poor sperm motility may be caused by antibodies
clinging to the sperm tail and thus interfering with forward mo-
tion. A test for antisperm antibodies can determine if this is the
case. The ability of sperm to actually penetrate an egg is not
assessed by the semen analysis, and problems with this important sperm function might occur even among normal-appearing
specimens. Sperm can be mixed together with specially pro-
cessed hamster eggs, and good sperm will fuse with the eggs,
while poor penetration of the eggs is a bad sign. A research
project in my laboratory is looking at the set of proteins contained
by sperm, since it appears that infertile sperm may be lacking
one or more important proteins. Work is in progress to see if a
protein test might be helpful for general use in the future.

Blood tests are often useful in evaluating infertile men. One
of the most useful blood tests is the FSH level. In Part I, I

described how FSH is made by the brain to stimulate the Sertoli cells in the testis. When the Sertoli cells are working properly, they make a substance called inhibin, which travels back to the brain and inhibits the production of FSH. This keeps FSH levels low. If the very important Sertoli cells within the testis are unhappy, they produce less inhibin and the FSH level rises. A very high FSH indicates a major fertility problem, whereas a normal level is reassuring. Other hormone tests may be useful as well, including testosterone and LH.

The most common abnormality seen on the semen analysis is a low sperm count, and if so, more often than not, the motility and percentage of normal-appearing sperm will be low as well. In other words, when the testicles put out low numbers of sperm, they also tend to make sperm of poor quality. What is a low sperm count? The average sperm concentration is roughly 60 to 80 million sperm per milliliter. However, we do not consider counts lower than this to be problematic until the numbers get as low as 20 million/ml. This number is somewhat arbitrary, since a count of 21 million/ml is practically the same as a count of 19 million/ml. Nevertheless, by definition, the fellow with a count of 19 million has an identifiable condition we called oligospermia (*oligo* = few), since it is less than 20 million/ml.

Picking a number such as 20 million sperm/ml is arbitrary because no one can say exactly what is the minimum number of sperm that a man needs to make a baby. Some men with very low numbers of sperm but with high quality (good motility and morphology) seem to have relatively little difficulty becoming fathers. And some men with fairly high numbers fail repeatedly to conceive. However, on balance, the more sperm available, the better the chances. Below a certain threshold the chances of a pregnancy occurring within a reasonable period of time diminish considerably.

Remember that fertility is a probability game. Only a fraction of the sperm entering the vagina make it into the cervix, and only a fraction of those make it through the cervical mucus into the uterus. Once inside the uterus the sperm still have a considerable distance to go up the tubes to meet the egg and interact with it in such a way that fertilization can take place. Men with sperm concentrations around 30 million will generally achieve a pregnancy, but it may take a longer time than usual. Men with concentrations of 20 million or less may also achieve a pregnancy without help, but the chances of this happening are reduced and diminish further as the numbers drop. These are the men who are usually referred for help.

■ VARICOCELE

One of the most common treatable causes of male infertility is a curious condition called varicocele. Varicocele refers to varicose veins within the scrotum. When a man stands up, he may feel something like a bag of worms above and behind his testicle, although this can be difficult to feel if the veins are not very large. Straining makes these veins stand out even more, and they will usually disappear when he lies down. Varicoceles are caused by missing or poorly functioning valves in the veins leading to the testicles, which normally act to prevent gravity from pulling blood downward. Most men with varicoceles are completely unaware of it, as it usually causes no discomfort. Although a very large varicocele may cause some men to have an annoying heaviness in their scrotum, there is otherwise no reason to pay much attention to a varicocele unless there is a fertility problem.

Many men have varicoceles. In one study, varicoceles were detected in 15 percent of army recruits. Most men with varicoceles are fertile, and it is not uncommon to find varicoceles among men who desire a vasectomy after completing their families. Why then should anyone think varicocele contributes to infertility if it is so common, even among fertile men?

One reason is that a high percentage of men seen at infertility centers with an abnormal semen analysis have varicoceles, up to 50 percent in some studies. And it turns out that when a varicocele is repaired, most men who had an abnormal semen analysis beforehand will have significant improvement. So there is no question that varicoceles may cause reversible infertility in some men.

But why should a varicose vein have anything to do with fertility? To understand this, I need to explain some more anatomy. Varicoceles almost always appear on the left, although they may also be accompanied by a right-sided varicocele. This preference for the left side is likely related to the asymmetry of the veins in the body. The vein from the left testicle drains into the left kidney vein, but on the right side the vein drains directly into the inferior vena cava, the biggest vein in the body. It is likely that there is higher pressure on the left side because of this arrangement. This higher pressure may overcome the valves in the testicular veins, and blood can then fill these veins backward to the testis when a man stands up. This blood flowing backward from the level of the kidney has been warmed by the body, and when the veins fill up, the testicles are then exposed to higher temperatures than usual. This exposure to heat is the leading explanation for how varicoceles impair fertility.

It is well established that the testicles require a cooler temperature than the rest of the body in order to produce sperm. This is why we have a scrotum, to keep the jewels cool. Testicles that fail to descend into the scrotum do not produce sperm. This infertility effect on the testicle appears to be due entirely to the higher temperature in the abdomen. The normal temperature difference between the body and the scrotum is only three to four degrees centigrade. It turns out that when a man with a varicocele stands up, the temperature in the scrotum goes up, but in a man without a varicocele the scrotal temperature decreases, presumably because the testicles hang farther away from the warm body. The temperature goes up with a varicocele because the warm blood from around the kidney descends rapidly through the veins into the scrotum where it surrounds and heats the testicles. When a varicocele is repaired, the temperature pattern returns to normal.

This association between temperature and varicocele does

not prove that this is the mechanism by which varicocele may interfere with normal fertility, but it does seem reasonable. I have been very interested in the effects of temperature on the testis, and current work in my laboratory is focused on the changes seen when testicular tissue is exposed to warmer temperatures. I suspect that a varicocele may diminish the fertility potential in any man, but most men have considerable reproductive reserves and it has minimal impact. For those men beginning with only moderate fertility, a varicocele may reduce sperm quality to the point that fertility becomes unlikely.

Surgical repair of a varicocele is a fairly straightforward procedure. The goal is to divide the veins carrying the excessively warm blood to the testis. An incision is made in the groin, like a hernia incision, and the veins are identified, cut, and tied. Some urologists prefer to use a higher incision. I like to use an operating microscope to be sure that I have tied off even the tiniest branches of veins, which otherwise might swell following the operation and act just like the original varicocele. The procedure takes approximately one hour, after which you go home. There is mild to moderate discomfort for several days around the incision.

Doctors are experimenting with new treatments for varicoceles. These include use of a laparoscope, or internal operating telescope, to tie off the offending veins through a puncture hole made in the abdomen. The theoretical advantage is that recovery will be quicker than with a regular incision. It is also possible to block the veins with X-ray guidance by passing a long, thin tube through the larger veins in the body and placing plugs in the veins leading to the testicles. Time will tell if these techniques offer any real advantages. For the time being, I have been very satisfied with my own microsurgical technique and results.

Success rates have varied, but generally one can expect that 50 to 70 percent of men with abnormal semen analysis and varicocele will have significant improvement in count, motility, or morphology. Pregnancy rates for couples who have no other known fertility problems are in the 30 to 50 percent range. The reason that pregnancy rates do not match improvement rates in the semen analysis is that other unrecognized problems may exist, particularly in the female partner. One reason that sperm quality does not improve in everyone is that there may be irreversible damage from the varicocele. In general, though, I am always pleased to find a varicocele in a man with an abnormal semen analysis, since it is a treatable problem with a good chance for improvement.

Not infrequently I will see a man who has already had his varicocele repaired without benefit. I examine these men very closely to see if they might still have a varicocele, perhaps one on the other side. Sometimes the size of a varicocele is reduced by surgery but it is still present. Since the diagnosis depends on the sensitivity of the doctor's fingers and how aggressively he looks for the varicocele in the examining room, many small varicoceles can be missed. If the semen analysis does not improve after surgery and there is still a varicocele present of any size, then I believe it is worthwhile to treat the varicocele again. I will often use the X-ray technique for repeat varicoceles to avoid operating through old scar tissue.

■ INFECTIONS AND INFERTILITY

Infections can certainly cause problems with male fertility. With genital infections one naturally thinks of gonorrhea or syphilis, but more commonly it is bacteria with such odd names as mycoplasma or ureaplasma that are the culprits when it comes to infertility. These bacteria may live quietly within the male genital tract, usually the urethra, without causing any obvious symptoms. The diagnosis is usually made by culture of the semen when the physician notices an increased number of white blood cells in the ejaculate, or if the sperm clump together. Treatment with antibiotics can be very effective. Occasionally, more troublesome bacteria are to blame, although these generally do cause symptoms, such as a discharge from the penis.

Albert came to me with a challenging problem of infertility due to infection. Albert was an engineering consultant who was born with a severe bladder disorder. As a child he had had his bladder removed, and the urine was diverted into a small opening on his lower abdominal wall, where it drains into a bag. Albert has sex and ejaculates normally, since the prostate, seminal vesicles, and urethra are all present. However, a semen analysis revealed that his sperm would stick together in big clumps, which is called agglutination. This can be a sign of infection. Albert also has a small amount of creamy drainage on his undershorts daily. He was treated elsewhere by several physicians with standard antibiotics without success. One doctor tried to wash the sperm and then perform artificial insemination. Nothing worked.

I obtained cultures on Albert's sperm, and our hospital laboratory found an unusual and particularly difficult bacteria. This bacteria is resistant to most antibiotics taken orally, and when it is found in the lungs or urine, patients generally need to be hospitalized for intravenous antibiotics.

I gave Albert a prescription for one of the newest oral antibiotics that often does work for this bacteria. At the end of the month his semen analysis was perfect. No agglutination at all. Since his count and motility were otherwise perfectly normal, I was optimistic for Albert and told him to call me when his wife was pregnant. Two months later came the happy news.

Other infections can also cause infertility in men, although antibiotics are not the solution. In some men infection can cause scarring of the testicles or of the tubes long after the infection has been treated. Gonorrhea is one such bacteria, and chlamydia is another. The most common place where scarring occurs is in the delicate epididymis. Usually this is noticed only if the scarring has affected both sides, since if one side is unaffected, the chances are good that a man will be normally fertile. On examination the epididymis may feel thickened and enlarged. No sperm will be seen on the semen analysis. Many of these men will do well by having a microsurgical connection made between the portion of the epididymis before the blockage and the open vas deferens beyond the scarring.

■ "Shooting Blanks"

The absence of any sperm in the ejaculate is called azoospermia. This may occur for various reasons, such as the scarring from infection I described above. Other possibilities, however, are that the testicles are not making any mature sperm, or the sperm are transported backward into the bladder during ejaculation.

Barry came to see me because he had concerns about his ability to father children. He explained that when he ejaculated, he would only occasionally see fluid come out the tip of his penis. During childhood Barry had an operation performed on the opening of his bladder because of recurrent bladder infections. Barry's examination was normal, but urine obtained following ejaculation was loaded with sperm. Barry had retrograde ejaculation, in which the semen travels into the bladder instead of out the tip of the penis. Since the sperm are washed out with the next urination, this is not a worrisome condition, and Barry needed no treatment at that time. Two years later Barry was married. I prescribed medication to help close the opening of the bladder, he developed partial forward ejaculation, and his wife became pregnant three months later.

If a normal amount of fluid is present but there are no sperm, the question is whether the sperm are blocked from coming out or are not being manufactured properly. The level of FSH in the blood is a good clue, since a high level of this hormone indicates a severe problem in the testicular machinery. If it is normal, or close to normal, then it is time to do a biopsy of the testis to see whether mature sperm are being formed.

Interpretation of the biopsy is straightforward in these cases. Either there is completely normal sperm production and development, indicating that there must be a blockage (since if they are being made but not getting out, there is no other possibility);

or they are being made but never mature properly; or they are not being produced in the first place. Some men have a condition diagnosed by biopsy called Sertoli-cell-only syndrome. Remember that the Sertoli cells are the nurse cells that help the sperm to develop, but the Sertoli cells never become sperm themselves. In this condition, no germ cells exist, only Sertoli cells. How this happens is unclear, but may be due to an accident of birth in which the germ cells never appeared, or perhaps they were wiped out by a silent infection.

If no mature sperm are seen on the biopsy, or no germ cells are seen, then there is no possible treatment. It is not possible to transplant germ cells from someone else into the testis. Even if it were possible, the genetic material would be from the germ cell donor, so that it would really not be biologically different from simply using sperm from a donor.

Azoospermia and a normal testis biopsy indicate an obstruction somewhere, and both sides must be affected (there should be sperm present in the ejaculate if only one side is obstructed). The most common cause for this is epididymitis, a not uncommon infection affecting the epididymis and the testicles. Epididymitis causes pain, swelling, and often fever. Although epididymitis is usually well treated with antibiotics and rest, there may be irreversible scarring of the delicate tubes within the epididymis resulting in a permanent blockage. If this occurs on both sides, a man will be azoospermic and sterile.

Fortunately for some, microsurgical techniques have advanced to the point that men with bilateral obstruction due to epididymitis have a reasonable chance of undergoing reconstructive surgery. The sperm can then bypass the segment of epididymis with the scarring and travel directly through the vas to the urethra with ejaculation. Pregnancy rates, however, are no greater than 20 to 30 percent, due to several factors, including the technical difficulty of the procedure, and impairment of the testis from long-standing obstruction. Nevertheless, many successes do occur, allowing couples with no hope otherwise to achieve a pregnancy naturally. These procedures should be performed by urologists who are experienced microsurgeons in order to have a reasonable hope for success.

A new treatment is now available for some men with azoospermia. Men born without the vas deferens have no way to get sperm out of the penis with ejaculation. This condition is called congenital absence of the vas deferens, or CAV. Men born with CAV were previously treated with an ingenious device called an artificial spermatocele. A spermatocele is a cyst of the epididymis containing sperm that forms naturally in some men. An artificial spermatocele was devised as a pouch that was surgically attached to the epididymis of men with CAV, with the hope that sperm would enter into this sac, and the sac could then be punctured by a needle through the skin. Sperm could then be withdrawn and used for insemination. Success rates have been extremely poor, due to technical considerations such as scarring of these extremely fine tubules. The use of alloplastic spermatoceles is now mainly of historical interest.

However, it is now possible to achieve pregnancies in some cases by puncturing the epididymis in a minor procedure and withdrawing sperm in great enough numbers so that fertilization of the wife's eggs can take place in a glass dish, called in vitro fertilization (IVF). The great advantage is that fertilization can be achieved with a relatively low number of sperm, such as those withdrawn from the blind-ending epididymis of men with CAV. This surgical extraction of sperm from the epididymis, combined with IVF, is also proving to be beneficial for other causes of obstructed tubes.

■ OTHER ASPECTS OF MALE INFERTILITY

Often there is no obvious reason why a man's sperm quality should be poor. The FSH may be normal or high, the testicles may be normal or somewhat small and soft, but there is nothing in the man's history to explain his problem, and no varicocele is present. These men fall into a group called idiopathic (cause is unknown) oligospermia. To say that there is still a lot to be learned about male infertility is one of the great understatements in medicine. However, research in the field is expanding, and I suspect we will have many more answers and improved treatments over the next decade.

Some men with idiopathic oligospermia can be treated with a medication called clomiphene citrate. This medication is used primarily for women and acts as an anti-estrogen. Estrogen is commonly called a female hormone, but it is present in men in small quantities, in critical areas such as the brain. It appears that the "male hormone" testosterone acts within the brain by first being converted to estrogen. An anti-estrogen makes the brain believe that there is less estrogen and testosterone around, and so it does its best to bring testosterone levels up to par by increasing the secretion of LH from the pituitary. LH then promotes further production of testosterone by the testis. This increased production of testosterone is thought to be the mechanism by which some men, perhaps as many as 30 percent, improve their sperm production while on clomiphene.

A small number of men appear to be infertile as a result of antibodies to their sperm. The antibodies stick to the sperm and interfere with its function, generally by interfering with swimming. Antibodies are part of the body's immune system, which is designed to fight foreign material such as viruses or bacteria. In order to do so it must be able to distinguish between self and nonself material. As discussed previously, the immune system is prevented from identifying sperm as foreign material by the blood-testis barrier. When this barrier breaks down, perhaps by infection or injury, antibodies can be formed against sperm.

Various treatments for antisperm antibodies have been proposed, including the use of steroids, which suppress the immune system. I tend to see antibodies as a sign of a system gone awry rather than as a specific cause of infertility by themselves. Washing the sperm to rid them of surface antibodies, then performing intrauterine insemination, is the usual approach to this problem.

■ Artificial Insemination and In Vitro Fertilization (IVF)

Some men may go through an extensive evaluation without finding an obvious cause for their poor sperm quality. If no specific problem can be identified, there can be no specific treatment. There are still several treatments for the couple, however, which attempt to maximize the chances of pregnancy given the limited number of sperm available. The simplest of these is called artificial insemination, or intrauterine insemination (IUI).

With intrauterine insemination a man ejaculates into a laboratory jar and the sperm are then washed free of the surrounding seminal fluid. The best sperm are then selected for placement within the uterine cavity. This selection process is rather clever. The sperm are first placed in a gentle fluid with an energy source so that they can swim freely. The test tube containing the sperm and fluid is then placed in a centrifuge, which packs the sperm into the bottom of the test tube. The test tube is then left standing for a time. As the good sperm begin to swim, many of them will rise from the bottom of the test tube, while the "poor swimmers" continue to lie at the bottom. The top layer of fluid soon contains the best sperm, and this layer is then removed.

Once this is done, the doctor takes the fluid and places it directly within the partner's uterus with a small tube, like a straw. The timing is crucial to have any hope of success, which means that this must be done just as the woman is ovulating. Sometimes the gynecologist will have the woman take medications that encourage the ovary to release more than the usual single egg, so that the odds of success are increased on the woman's side as well. Intrauterine insemination takes only a few minutes for the woman, and there should be only a twinge of discomfort. This is a very reasonable step for couples to take for a variety of causes of infertility, including male infertility. It is simple, safe, and effective for many couples.

If IUI fails after a series of attempts, or there are certain problems on the woman's side such as blocked tubes, or the man's sperm quality is really poor, the next step might be in vitro fertilization (IVF). *In vitro* literally means "in glass," and the term *IVF* refers to the fact that in this technique the sperm and egg are incubated together in a glass dish so that fertilization can take place. In other words, the embryo begins its journey outside the human body. Once fertilization has occurred, the embryo is placed within the womb just as with IUI.

IVF has been a tremendous advance in the treatment of infertility, allowing many couples to achieve pregnancy who were previously unable to do so. But there are several drawbacks and limitations. The most important is that IVF is a long way from being successful for everyone. Success rates vary from center to center, but a 25 percent success rate is considered fairly good. Three out of four couples who go through the IVF process will still be unsuccessful. Another problem for many is cost. In many states health insurers do not cover IVF, and because it is so high tech, it tends to be expensive, often costing upwards of $10,000. These costs place IVF out of the price range of many couples. Still, IVF may be a good step for a couple with a male fertility problem.

Micromanipulation is a promising technique that places one or more individual sperm right next to the egg membrane, beneath the protective covering of its shell, the zona pellucida. Normally, sperm must penetrate this shell before contacting the egg. Micromanipulation thus removes a major obstacle from the sperm, like placing a jewel thief directly within the room containing the safe without needing to deal with the guards and the alarm system. Micromanipulation requires fancy equipment to hold the microscopic egg in place, while needles much finer than anything you could see with your eye pierce the zona pellucida under the microscope and deposit a few sperm.

A handful of fertility centers around the country have reported success with this technique for men who had failed at everything else, generating considerable excitement. Although the number of successes has been very few, as techniques improve this may be an important treatment for male infertility in the future.

■ END OF THE LINE—WHAT TO DO?

The treatment of infertility does not always work out. There may have been a period of hope with multiple tries of IUI or IVF, or months on medications, or surgery. Some men may have been told right away that they were completely sterile and there was no way that they could ever be the genetic father of a child. What to do?

For most men and their partners this is a critical moment in their lives. As children we fantasize about growing up and what it would be like to be an adult. For many, these fantasies involve thoughts about what it would be like to be a father, how one would act similar to or different from one's parents. Few individuals are prepared for the idea that they may be infertile, and so the information comes as a shock.

At the end of the line, when there is nothing more to be done, or a decision has been made to try no further, there may be a variety of emotions, including anger, frustration, and disappointment. However, foremost among these is grief. This grief is for the children hoped for who will never arrive. It is for the parent one had hoped to become and for the anticipated family that was not meant to be. This period of loss and sadness places a tremendous burden on a marriage. Unless there is honest and open talk between the partners, the relationship may founder. Individual or couples counseling can be extremely helpful to keep the demons of guilt, resentment, and anger out on the table where they can be addressed, instead of letting them fester internally and damage an otherwise loving relationship.

Although some couples may choose to live their lives child-free, other options are available. If male infertility is the problem and the woman has no medical conditions interfering with her fertility, then donor insemination may be a good solution. Sperm from an anonymous fertile man are used for artificial insemination during the ovulatory period so that the woman can become pregnant and go through a normal pregnancy. Although the male partner is not the genetic or biological father, by providing emotional support during the pregnancy and by being involved in the process, most men find it quite natural to consider themselves a parent in every sense of the word.

Many couples have concerns about donor insemination. Who is the actual donor, for instance, and how can we know that he doesn't have some disease such as AIDS or a genetic defect? Because of these concerns, it is important to have donor insemination performed through an established program, where thorough screening of donors is performed. Donors are often students and must be in good health without a family history of genetic defects. To guard against the possibility of transmitting infections, the sperm samples are frozen and the donors undergo regular testing, including blood tests for AIDS. The frozen sperm samples are quarantined for at least six months and are released for use only if blood tests still show no trace of AIDS or other diseases.

Donor insemination may not be the right solution for every couple, and they may then choose adoption. Adoption has its own set of benefits and problems, but is clearly the right solution for many couples. A large number of reputable adoption agencies exist, and though it may take time and money, the bottom line is that couples who want to be parents can do so. Since the issues involved in deciding what is right for any given couple are so complex and emotional, I think it is extremely important to talk things over with a therapist or counselor before proceeding with adoption or donor insemination.

Often it is difficult to know where to find help. One of the best consumer advocacy groups is the national organization called Resolve, which is devoted to supporting and educating people with infertility. This group has the resources to steer individuals and couples toward the professionals and information they need to make informed, careful choices about their lives. If you are having problems with infertility, I encourage you to get the help and support you need, from your partner, your physician, and from organizations such as Resolve.

CHAPTER 3

TESTICULAR PROBLEMS

■ PAIN

Pain in the testicles is a universal experience for men. For most, it is one that is experienced rarely, and for no more than an instant or two. The testicles hang in a fairly precarious position, presumably to allow them to function better in a cooler environment, as discussed previously. They are thus exposed to the vagaries of modern society, including tight underwear and tight pants. Few youths and athletes fail to experience an inadvertent projectile landing in their true midsection. Aside from the pain of a direct blow to the scrotum, however, there are other types of testicular pain that may be medically important.

Most men experience intermittent twinges of pain in the scrotum that come and go without any warning and generally last no more than a few seconds. It is not unusual for me to see men with this problem, particularly after a friend has had some major medical problem somewhere in the genital region. If a man has suffered any sort of genital problem, he is then much more likely to focus on the transient aches and pains that would previously have been ignored. If pain in the testicles last less than a minute or two and then disappears, it is unlikely that there is anything to worry about. On the other hand, persistent pain lasting minutes to hours is another subject altogether and requires medical attention.

Many people associate pain with cancer, and this holds true for pain in the testicles. However, this association is not usually correct. Although testis cancer is occasionally discovered after a man experiences pain in the testicles, it is usually discovered as a painless lump. Pain generally indicates swelling, infection, or poor blood supply to the testis.

Pain that comes on gradually and builds to an unpleasant crescendo is usually due to an infection or inflammation of the testis or the epididymis. This is called epididymitis if the epididymis is affected the most, and orchitis if the testis is affected most. These can cause scarring of the tubules and infertility, as I mentioned before. If untreated, it can also progress to an abscess, and on rare occasions removal of the testis is necessary to cure the infection. More commonly, epididymitis is treated successfully with antibiotics. If caught early enough in its course, oral antibiotics are fine. If the infection has progressed or is severe, it may be necessary to hospitalize the man so that he may receive intravenous antibiotics.

Alan was a young man in his early twenties who was admitted to the hospital with fever and severe testicular pain. The day before he had helped his friend push his disabled car to the service station, and later that evening he began to feel mild discomfort in his left testicle. By the next morning he was so miserable with pain that he could barely walk. His girlfriend brought him in to the emergency room.

Alan looked quite ill. His temperature was 103, and his heart was beating rapidly. The left testicle was swollen to twice its normal size, and the overlying skin was bright red. The testicle was slightly tender, but as soon as I touched the epididymis, he hollered with pain. Alan had acute epididymitis and was treated with intravenous antibiotics for several days in the hospital. His fever came down, and the tenderness in the testicle was almost gone by the time he left the hospital. It would take another month before the testicle returned to its normal size.

Straining can cause epididymitis because it produces high pressures within the urethra, and a few drops of urine may be forced down the tubes toward the epididymis and testicle. Urine can be very irritating, and if there are any bacteria present, they may infect the delicate epididymis. I suspect this is what happened to Alan.

■ TORSION

Another important cause of testicular pain is called torsion. Torsion is a twist of the spermatic cord, which provides the blood supply to the testicle. Occasionally a testicle will twist as much as twice around, squeezing off its blood supply. This causes excruciating pain. It is not difficult to convince someone with testicular torsion to go to the hospital.

Sometimes a man will have experienced milder versions of this pain in the past that resolved after several minutes, which probably represented a mild twist, and a subsequent untwisting. Usually the pain of torsion comes on suddenly and does not stop until the twist is undone. Nausea, vomiting, or low abdominal pain may occur with the testicular pain. There is approximately four to six hours grace before the testis suffers irreversible damage from a lack of blood.

The treatment for torsion is an operation to untwist the testicle and its blood supply. The affected testicle and its partner on the other side are both sutured to the wall of the scrotum so that they can never twist again. Sometimes the testicle can be untwisted in the emergency room, or it may untwist by itself. Men who are lucky enough to have the torsion go away by itself must still have surgery at some point to fix the testicles, since they are at risk for having torsion again. Some men seem prone to torsion by the way their testicles are attached to surrounding tissues. Their testicles hang more loosely within the scrotum and are thus unusually free to rotate.

Most cases of torsion occur in childhood, and it seems likely that some occur even before birth. A testis missing in a newborn may be either undescended or absent from torsion. In an infant it may be difficult to determine if he is in pain, and if so, what is the source. Infants with testicular swelling or scrotal discoloration should be seen immediately by a physician.

■ Lumps, Bumps, and Testis Cancer

We hear it on radio and television, and we read it in magazines and books: feeling a lump somewhere in the body can be a sign of cancer. It is therefore alarming for a man to examine his testicles, since the whole scrotal area feels lumpy and bumpy. Most of the time these lumps and bumps are part of the normal anatomy, but a number of benign conditions can also be felt as a mass or make the scrotum look enlarged. And yes, once in a great while a mass in the scrotum can be a cancer.

Eugene was a fifty-year-old man who had noticed a lump in the right side of his sac for three months. It did not seem to be growing in size, but it was also not shrinking. When Eugene felt the right side of his scrotum, it felt as if he had two testicles on that side, one atop the other. He had no pain in the area, not even when he squeezed it.

When I examined Eugene, the right side of his scrotum was clearly enlarged. I could feel a normal testicle with a somewhat firm mass just above it. I turned down the lights and shined a flashlight against the back of Eugene's scrotum. When I placed the light behind the testis, the solid testis blocked the light and created a dark area. I then placed the light behind the mass, and the light shined through with a deep red as if it were shining directly through skin. This told me the mass was filled with clear fluid.

Eugene had a benign condition called a spermatocele, which is a cyst of the epididymis, usually containing sperm. Although they can be bothersome if they grow to a large size, spermatoceles otherwise require no treatment. Most men are greatly relieved to learn they do not have a malignancy. The key to the diagnosis was shining the light against the mass in a darkened room, called transillumination. Solid things, such as testicles and tumors, block the light, whereas fluid-filled cysts let the light pass right through. The red color comes from the blood in the skin.

Another benign condition that is also quite common is called a hydrocele, which consists of a fluid collection around the testicle itself. These can grow very large and may be mistaken for a large hernia. They sometimes follow injuries to the testicle from trauma or infections. Hydroceles also do not require treatment unless their size interferes with daily activities.

A more worrisome "lump" story came to my attention several years ago. The nurse in the occupational-health office of the hospital called me, quite concerned about a twenty-eight-year-old maintenance man she had just seen, named Jeff. He claimed that he had been hit in the genital area by a segment of vent duct while working that day. When the nurse examined Jeff, his scrotum did not have the appearance of a recent injury. However, his left scrotum was tremendously enlarged with a hard mass that was not tender. She questioned him further about the timing of the swelling, since the story did not fit for an acute injury. Jeff admitted there might have been some swelling for several days. I asked to see Jeff right away.

Jeff walked easily into my office. He was a healthy single man who had never been sick a day in his life. He told me the same story he had told the nurse, about how he had walked into the ventilation duct lying on a workbench, striking him in the scrotal area. On examination, the left side of his scrotum was the size of a grapefruit. There was no sign of recent injury, such as bruising or swelling. The mass in the scrotum was hard, and when I tried to shine a light through it, it would not transilluminate. This indicated it was not simply a benign collection of fluid such as a hydrocele or spermatocele. There was no doubt in my mind that this was a testicular cancer, and that it had been there for quite some time, probably growing for months.

I asked Jeff how long he had noticed the swelling. "A few days," he answered. I pushed him a little harder. Any chance this had been present longer than that? "Maybe a couple of weeks, definitely no longer than that." I told him I was very concerned that it was cancer. He would need to have his testis removed. Blood tests and an X ray of the testis called an ultrasound would need to be performed. Jeff would be hospitalized that day, and I would perform his operation the next day. Jeff did not understand. He refused to believe this was a cancer. "It's from getting banged there today, Doc," he insisted.

People are funny when it comes to illness. I am sure it is an oversimplification, but it seems to me that people can be divided into two groups based on how they respond emotionally to a potential problem. The first group always thinks the worst, which usually means that every ache and pain might indicate cancer. The second group tends to deny the significance of key symptoms such as the development of severe chest tightness with activity, or the growth of a huge mass in the scrotum. My impression is that men are most often deniers. Certainly Jeff fell into this group.

Deniers deny for at least two reasons. The first is that men, in particular, are taught not to complain about physical injuries, that this constitutes being weak or a sissy. This attitude can be carried too far, of course. There are appropriate times to complain, and it is foolish to be quiet about a potential health problem that may be easily treated.

The second reason is that the idea of having a problem such as a cancer may be so frightening that one is afraid to have one's fears confirmed. Many people do not understand or believe that, for the most part, cancers are treatable illnesses. The vast majority of cancers are completely curable if detected early. Indeed, the purpose of increasing public awareness about cancer is to get people into the doctor's office in time to have a cancer cured. Nevertheless, a large number of otherwise intelligent people still feel that if they come down with a cancer, there is no point in seeing the doctor, since they are already as good as dead.

I wanted Jeff to have his surgery right away. He had clearly put off seeing anyone about the mass in his scrotum for a considerable length of time, and I did not want him to get cold feet and postpone his treatment any longer. Even the way he sought medical attention underscored how much difficulty he had facing up to this problem. After the ultrasound test confirmed a large testicular mass characteristic of cancer, I spoke with Jeff again. I told him the cancer had likely been there for as long as several months. Was he sure he hadn't noticed any swelling or lumps during that time? Two weeks at most, he replied, still arguing that the swelling was due to his injury that day. Jeff returned the next day for his surgery. When the nurse was asking her routine preoperative questions, she asked how long the mass had been there. "About a month," he answered.

The surgery went well, despite the enormous size of the tumor. The incision for tumors of the testicle is made in the groin, not the scrotum, so that the entire spermatic cord including blood vessels and lymphatic channels can be removed together with the testicle. An artificial testicle, called a testicular prosthesis, can be placed in the scrotum to give the appearance and feel of having two testicles, and Jeff chose to have this done. He went home the next day, with moderate soreness in the area of his incision, which improved over the next week.

Testis cancer comes in two main types, only one of which is sensitive to radiation. Jeff had the nonsensitive kind. His X rays of the abdomen and chest and his blood tests did not indicate any spread of disease. However, because X rays cannot detect microscopic amounts of disease in the lymph nodes, it is often necessary to do an operation in which the lymph nodes in the back part of the abdomen are removed for microscopic examination. I performed this operation on Jeff several weeks later. The lymph nodes showed no tumor. This was an excellent report and meant that Jeff needed no further treatment other than close observation in case the cancer reappeared in the future. Jeff showed up for his first postoperative appointment, then missed all his next visits despite reminders from the office.

Approximately one year later Jeff came to the emergency room with trouble breathing. His X rays showed tumor in the lungs. He was treated with chemotherapy. His hair fell out, he lost weight, he developed terrible diarrhea. The chemotherapy ended and Jeff went home. Three years later, Jeff is back at work, sometimes keeping his appointments, sometimes not. There is no more evidence for cancer. We almost lost him, but he is now cured.

Jeff's story is important because it demonstrates that even if a lump in the testis turns out to be cancer, there is every likelihood that it can be treated and cured. However, proper treatment depends on a close working relationship between physician and patient. Jeff almost died because he was so reluctant to follow through with his doctor's recommendations. The metastases could have been picked up earlier by X rays or blood tests and could have been treated more easily at that time.

Testis cancer differs from other cancers in many ways, but there are also similarities between cancers that allow doctors to give them one general name. Cancer occurs when normal cells become altered and begin to divide continuously. This results in a growing mass, which is why cancers often appear as lumps. Cancers cause problems in two main ways: by compressing or invading nearby normal tissues as the tumor grows, and by the shedding of tumor cells into the bloodstream or lymphatics, which then spread to other parts of the body. This spread of cancer is called metastasis.

Testis cancers tend to spread early, which is bad, but the path of their spread is predictable, which is good. Approximately 40 percent of testis tumors have metastasized at the time of diagnosis. Since the path of spread is so predictable, it is possible to look in a few specific areas with X rays to see if there are any metastases. This also permits a logical stepwise approach to treatment, which has certainly contributed to the high success rate in treating this disease.

The two main types of testis cancer are called seminoma and, for lack of a better word, nonseminoma. Seminoma is the most common single type of testis tumor, occurring in roughly 40 percent of cases. The nonseminoma group is actually composed of several different types of tumors. The main reason for lumping the nonseminomas together is that they respond to therapy in a similar way. Namely, seminoma is extremely sensitive to radiation, and the nonseminomas are not. They require chemotherapy because of their resistance to treatment with radiation.

The treatment of testis cancer is one of the great success stories of medicine over the last twenty years. Before that time seminoma was a fairly treatable tumor, with radiation, but the other tumors offered a poor prognosis. The advent of effective chemotherapy brought about extremely high cure rates for nonseminomas for the first time. It is now rare to lose a patient like Jeff.

Testis cancer is the most common cancer among men in their twenties and thirties, however it is still an uncommon disease. Young boys may also develop testis tumors. Testis cancer strikes at a time when many men still have a sense of invulnerability and immortality, and the diagnosis cuts them emotionally right down to the quick. Not only must one confront the specter of death from a malignant disease but there are also issues of being less than whole in an area of considerable concern.

In a study examining the emotional impact of testis cancer on a group of men who had been cured of their illness, Drs. Susan Edbril and Patricia Rieker learned that many of these men had gone out of their way to perform acts to affirm their masculinity. One man performed a triathlon shortly after completing debilitating chemotherapy. Another engaged in as many sexual encounters as he could. It is obvious that a severe illness affecting the testicles can affect one's self-image in profound ways.

CHAPTER 4

THE TESTICULAR SELF-EXAM

■ Although testis cancer is quite uncommon, it is important for all men, particularly those between the ages of eighteen and thirty-five, to be able to perform a testicular self-exam. This is because cancer of the testis usually causes no pain or discomfort and is discovered as a hard lump. In the vast majority of cases an abnormality will prove to be nothing serious, and in the rare case where a cancer is found, it is more likely to be cured if diagnosed early.

It helps to do the exam in a warm location so that the scrotum is relaxed and the testicles hang down. A warm bath is an ideal place for the exam. The first thing to know is that the testicles hang down from the body by a thick cord, called the spermatic cord, which carries the blood vessels and vas deferens. By gently placing thumb and forefinger together around the upper portion of the scrotum, you can slowly slide your fingers off to the side, allowing the structures of the cord to slip between your fingers. You may feel something similar to a thick guitar string in the cord, and this is the vas deferens.

Further below is the testicle itself. Through the skin you

should be able to feel a smooth surface to the front of the testis. Above, below, and behind the testis you might feel something lumpy or bumpy, soft or firm. This is the epididymis, and it is a completely normal structure. In some men it is easy to feel, and in others difficult. The normal testis is oval and smooth and feels much like a hard-boiled egg with the shell removed. The testis should be gently compressed, feeling for hard areas within it, or lumps that distort the smooth surface. It is good to compare one side to the other. If you feel anything that is worrisome to you, bring it to the attention of your doctor immediately. Even if your doctor tells you that everything is normal, this is helpful, since you now have a baseline that you know is all right, and any further changes merit close attention. I recommend performing a testicular exam once a month.

CHAPTER 5

IMPOTENCE

■ An impotent patient of mine who happens to be a doctor with a wonderful sense of humor told me this story. An older man walks into the doctor's office and says, "Doctor, when I was twenty years old my penis would get as hard as a steel rod. When I turned forty, I found that I could bend it a little bit. Now that I am sixty, I can bend it right back on itself. What I've learned from this is that as a man gets older, his hand strength increases dramatically." There is much truth hidden in this story. For example, the quality of men's erections deteriorate over time, so that even a perfectly functioning sixty-year-old is not likely to have quite the same rigidity he had thirty years previously, whether he recognizes the difference or not.

If a married man has sex with his wife on a regular basis without difficulty, it is unlikely that he would pay much attention to how rigid his penis becomes. The same man starting out in a new sexual relationship, however, may discover that his penile rigidity is not adequate to do what he would like to do. In the first case, there is likely to be a habitual way of having sex that does not place high demands on the penis, and intercourse is likely to be anxiety free. However, with a new partner, there may be a period of getting to know one another sexually when lovemaking is not so smooth, and this may require more penile rigidity to succeed at penetration. The point is that an erection that is adequate for one situation may not be adequate for another. Impotence is often not an absolute lack of erections, but rather a lack of adequate rigidity. The diagnosis really depends on a functional question—is the rigidity good enough for sex? Of course there are men who have lost the ability to achieve any rigidity at all, and others who develop excellent rigidity, but only for a brief moment. These men fill out the spectrum of what we call impotence or erectile dysfunction.

To review the anatomy and some of the processes leading to erection, recall that there are two cylinders within the penis called the corpora cavernosa, which fill with blood to produce an erection. A tough sheath called the tunica albuginea surrounds each of the corpora cavernosa so that as the cylinders fill, they first reach their maximum distension, and then the pressure rises to the level of the pressure in the arteries. This produces rigidity. In order to maintain stiffness, the blood must be trapped effectively within the corpora cavernosa. During sexual arousal the brain sends messages to the muscle fibers within the penis that govern the activity of the blood vessels, increasing the inflow of blood to the penis and activating the trapping mechanism. Sexual arousal is influenced by many factors, including state of mind, anxiety, smells, visual stimulation, touch, as well as the internal chemical environment of the brain, including adequate levels of testosterone. If inflow, outflow, nerve signals, and hormones are all okay, and the mind is willing, then an erection occurs. If any one of these is off, however, there will be a problem with erections.

Impotence is a remarkably common problem. Old data from Kinsey indicated that the prevalence of impotence increased with age and affected approximately 10 percent of men at age fifty, 20 percent at sixty, and 30 percent at seventy. Since most men are reluctant to discuss sex at all, let alone admit to something such as impotence, which might be perceived as a loss of their manhood, it is a safe bet that these figures grossly underestimate the problem. And impotence can affect men at all ages. Although the majority of men I see for erection problems are in their fifties and sixties, I have treated a large number of men in their twenties as well, some of whom developed difficulties as a teenager. As men reach their seventies, poor erections become the rule rather than the exception.

I have a recurring conversation in the office with mature patients. They will sit down, tell me about their problems with intercourse, then ask me if they are simply "too old" for sex. The answer, of course, is that no one is "too old" if he still has the desire. Although impotence becomes increasingly common with age, it does not follow that it should be considered a normal part of aging, any more than developing heart disease should be considered normal. We treat heart disease so that men can continue their daily activities, and likewise it makes good sense to treat impotence.

I believe a cultural attitude lies behind part of the question about being too old for sex. This attitude regards sex as some forbidden fruit, even within the confines of a marriage sanctioned by law and religion. Even after being married forty years, some men will admit that sex still feels like some delicious but naughty act they perform with their wives. The loss of erections then becomes similar to the teacher taking away the cards upon discovering the kids playing in the back row during class. You are upset the teacher took the cards away, but you know you should not have been playing in the first place.

But the analogy does not really hold up. Let's face it. Sex is one of the most basic human (and nonhuman) drives. For many couples, sex is not only a pleasurable activity but it may also be one of the few ways that affection is communicated within the relationship. The loss of erections for a man will often have an impact on his relationships as a whole, not to mention his sense of self, his sense of manhood. For these reasons, I think it is important for men to seek help when erection problems appear.

In the pages that follow I will describe the usual kinds of problems that occur, the way to diagnose the underlying condition, and the various treatments available today.

■ INADEQUATE INFLOW—ARTERIAL PROBLEMS

Bill was a healthy single man in his early thirties who was not currently in a relationship. Since his college days he had not been able to achieve a firm erection, although he was often able to have sex with a semihard erection after considerable stimulation. With masturbation his erections were no better. He remembered having normally firm erections as a teenager and had not had any problems with a girlfriend his freshman year in school. He was unaware of anything that might have happened to change the firmness of his erections. His physical examination was completely normal, and he seemed to be a solid, "both feet on the ground" sort of fellow.

Usually, a story of normal erections suddenly changing to poor erections indicates the acute onset of an illness, or more commonly some emotional event that prevents the man from becoming completely aroused or relaxed with sex. I wondered whether this might not be the case with Bill.

To see if Bill could achieve normal erections at a time when he was not focused on his problem, I performed a sleep study of his penis. This involves placing a small band around the penis before going to sleep, similar to a blood pressure cuff. The band is attached to a monitor the size of a small portable radio. During sleep, the device records the size and rigidity of the penis every minute. Men normally have four to eight erections each night, and these are easily demonstrated on the printout from the monitor by periods of increased penis size and increased rigidity. The anxiety that may be present during a sexual encounter and that may interfere with erections should be absent during sleep. If impotence is due to emotional factors, the sleep study should register normal penile rigidity. On the other hand, if there is a physical problem, then the sleep study should show poor erections.

Bill's sleep study was abnormal. It showed several erections, but with only moderate rigidity. Bill then underwent two tests to evaluate first his inflow, then his outflow. The test of the arteries showed that only reduced amounts of blood were able to travel into the penis. However, the ability to trap blood in the penis was completely normal. An X ray outlining the arteries to the penis was performed, and it showed a blockage of those arteries just under the pubic bone.

This blockage explained Bill's problem, and the likelihood was that Bill had suffered some sort of straddle injury, in which the arteries running under the pubic bone were injured by a blow or considerable pressure. Before I had a chance to describe his X rays, Bill volunteered that after thinking it over some more, he had had an accident that might be related. While skiing in college he had lost his balance and ended up going straight into a tree, with his legs winding up on opposite sides, just like in the cartoons. Although Bill was sore for several days, he had not needed medical attention and had put the accident out of his mind. His erections worsened several months later.

I told Bill that his X ray was completely consistent with the injury he described. Surgery to bypass the blocked arteries would have a good chance of success. However, Bill preferred for the time being to treat his impotence with injection of medication and has continued to do so with good results for the last two years. More on injections later.

The arteries carry blood to the penis, and men with inflow problems will either have to work strenuously to achieve rigidity or will be unable to get an erection at all. Young men with arterial blockages are most likely to have a story like Bill's, with an injury producing the blockage right under the pubic bone. Some evidence suggests that bicycle riders are at risk for impotence, since the narrow bicycle seat of serious cyclists puts pressure exactly at the point where the arteries cross under the bone. If you do a lot of cycling, it might be a good idea to pad your bicycle seat. If you are experiencing problems with erections, you should find another form of exercise.

More commonly, arterial problems causing impotence occur in men with atherosclerosis, or narrowing of the arteries. For many men (and women, too), this is a widespread process, affecting the blood vessels to the heart, brain, and legs among others. Men at risk for atherosclerosis include those with high blood pressure, diabetes, high cholesterol, and smokers. All of these, except certain forms of diabetes, are under one's personal control, through diet, medication, or behavioral changes, and in some cases controlling the underlying problem will help with the quality of erections as well.

■ FLAT TIRES AND SLOW LEAKS

Some men are able to achieve rigid erections, but within a short time they lose stiffness, so that they either cannot penetrate, or they cannot maintain enough rigidity to stay inside. This is often more embarrassing than a total lack of erections, since there is some initial promise, which is then frustrated. Men describe this as similar to a slow leak from a flat tire. What actually happens is that the penis fills normally with arterial blood, but the trapping mechanism malfunctions. Blood seeps out through the normal channels, but too early. The amount of blood coming into the penis cannot keep up with all the blood leaving, and the erection softens. When this venous leak, as it is called, is large enough, it is impossible to achieve any rigidity at all. If you are unable to maintain an erection under any circumstances, chances are you have a venous leak.

The veins that drain the corpora cavernosa run just inside the tough sheath. As the brain signals the penis to become firm, the arteries swell, increasing blood flow into the penis. Cushions of tissue within the penis expand against the veins, compressing them shut against the sheath. This diminishes the flow of blood out of the penis. After ejaculation the arteries shrink, and compression of the veins is relieved. This allows blood to flow through the veins out of the penis, and the penis becomes soft.

Venous leaks occur when the ability to compress these veins is reduced. If the cushions of tissue are stiff and cannot compress the veins adequately, then blood will continue to leave the penis. As the condition worsens, there will be difficulty maintaining an erection, and finally no erection at all. It turns out that the majority of cases of impotence are due to venous leaks.

The cause of the internal stiffness responsible for venous leaks is unknown. Diabetic men suffer from venous leaks as well as from arterial problems, and they have been shown to have increased stiffness of one of the main internal substances within the penis. In some cases where the penis has been injured, the body responds by forming scar tissue, which also is stiff, and incapable of compressing the internal penile veins. This results in a venous leak as well.

■ HORMONES AND IMPOTENCE

Testosterone is the hormone that governs sexual behavior in men. Testosterone is often called the male hormone, since it is made by the testicles and is present in high concentration in men, and in low concentration in women (small amounts are made by the adrenal glands, near the kidneys). Male animals deprived of testosterone will not participate in sexual activity when housed with a receptive female. However, electrical stimulation of the appropriate nerves or brain centers will produce a normal erection. This suggests that the main action of testosterone is on the brain, and that it affects what we call the sex drive or libido.

Irving was a fifty-five-year-old businessman who stepped into the office and immediately told me that he had come to see me only because his wife insisted he see a doctor. Over the last five years Irving and his wife had had sex no more than once every six months, always at his wife's insistence. His erections were not good anymore, he insisted. When we spoke some more, it turned out that Irving had little if any libido. "To tell the truth, Doctor, I could take it or leave it. And usually, I'd prefer to leave it." Irving no longer awakened with erections in the morning, and he took no notice of attractive women. He had no interest in masturbation. Other areas of his life were good, and he was feeling very well. However, his wife was concerned.

When I examined Irving, I noticed he had small, soft testicles. Blood tests on Irving came back as expected. His testosterone was quite low. I gave him several injections of testosterone, and I saw him two months later. He walked in with a big smile. "Everything's great," he said. He and his wife were back to having sex twice weekly, and they had even gone away for a weekend and "hardly got out of bed." Irving has continued on monthly injections and is very pleased. There was never anything wrong with the hydraulic system of his penis. The low testosterone had merely stalled the control center in his brain.

■ PSYCHOLOGICAL FACTORS

Sometimes a loss of libido signifies something other than low testosterone. For one thing, nearly all men who are impotent end up finding sexual encounters unpleasant, frustrating, and even embarrassing. They end up avoiding sexual situations. One man told me that he started staying up late watching television so that his wife would fall asleep and his inability to perform sexually would go unnoticed. After enough frustration, the mind makes a subconscious decision to extinguish all thoughts of sex so that further unpleasantness is avoided. Often, but not always, men can think back and recall whether their diminished interest in sex came before or after they developed trouble with erections. If it came afterward, this is a normal human reaction. If it came before, however, I wonder if the testosterone level is low, or if some emotional factors may be contributing to the problem.

Sex is such a complex issue that it is often extremely difficult to untangle all the psychological pieces that go into a man's attitude about himself as a sexual creature, and how he feels about others sexually. In the simplest instances it is easy enough to see how the mind may interfere with normal sexual functioning, but few situations are straightforward. The young, inexperienced man who is nervous about sex with a new partner has a good chance of failing to achieve a decent erection because of a discharge of adrenaline, which interferes with obtaining an erection. The situation is somewhat more complex in the man who finds himself unable to have sex with his wife ever since he witnessed the bloody birth of his child. The normally pleasurable thoughts of sex have been altered so that the vagina is now mentally associated with an emotionally traumatic event. Some cases of psychogenic impotence are easier to treat than others. Although I generally refer these cases to experienced therapists, occasionally I am comfortable making simple suggestions, which can be quite helpful.

A good example was Giuseppe, a construction worker in his fifties who complained of poor erections. When I asked him to describe what actually took place when he tried to have sex with his wife, he told me that when he initiated sex by kissing and touching his wife, she would begin to respond, but would then disengage and hop into the shower before she was ready to have intercourse. Over the last year, by the time she came out of the shower, Giuseppe no longer had an erection, and only occasionally was he able to achieve one again in order to have sex. I never inquired as to the temperature of the water, but his wife's actions had the effect of a cold shower on him.

To solve this particular puzzle, Giuseppe had to let his wife know that he found it frustrating for her to leave the bed when he was ready to have sex; and his wife needed to feel that she did not need to be freshly showered for Giuseppe to want to have intercourse with her. After Giuseppe and his wife talked things over, they had a more satisfying sexual relationship.

Diminished libido or poor erections may also indicate depression or emotional stress. A patient of mine is the owner of a small business who was unable to have sex during the week, but had no problem at all when he went away with his wife for the weekend. He admitted that when he tried to have sex during the week, his business worries found their way into his thoughts, and he quickly lost his erection.

An architect came to see me with a more complex situation. His erections had been of poor quality for some time, and he and his wife had not had sex in over three months. He had some vague desire for sex, but nothing like what it had been even a year earlier. Was he otherwise happy in the marriage? Yes. Were any stressful events occurring at work? No. Anything else that he thought might be contributing to his problem? No.

When it came time to arrange for a follow-up visit, he indicated that finding a time might be difficult since his father was dying of cancer in another state, and he would be traveling to take care of the arrangements at any time. It then also came out that his oldest child had been discovered using illegal drugs. This lovely man was overwhelmed with personal problems, but was not prepared to concede that they might be contributing to his sexual difficulties. While it is possible that there was a physical basis to his impotence, there would be no point in performing an elaborate medical evaluation until the emotional issues were addressed. He needed counseling and emotional support rather than a medical "fix."

Part of the elegant economy of most animals is that sexual activity diminishes when the organism is stressed. Rats undergoing experimental shock treatments, or other animals whose home environment has been destroyed by fire or flood, are not sexually active during the upheaval. This makes sense, since it would be a waste of energy and resources to care for newborns under hostile conditions threatening one's own survival. Humans are no different. During illness, one's libido is generally diminished. Emotional stress or depression may produce the same effect. When a depressed man complains of poor erections, the usual scenario is that his sex drive is low as well, which merely reflects the inner state of the man. Counseling or psychotherapy is often extremely helpful for these men, since the problem with their penis is no more than the tip of the iceberg.

Having said all this, it is important to stress that the vast majority of men who describe a long-standing progressive problem with erections have a physical rather than a psychological problem. This cannot be emphasized enough, since an attitude from the 1970s persists that impotence is primarily a psychological problem. The gurus of human sexuality from that time, Masters and Johnson, are largely responsible for this. At the time of their extensive studies of men with sexual difficulties, little was known about normal erections, and the ability to study erections was limited. The only physical causes for impotence recognized at the time were severe arterial disease in the blood vessels of the pelvis and low testosterone levels.

Much of Masters and Johnson's investigations were based on psychological profiles and questionnaires. Most men indicated that they had some negative feelings about sex, including frustration and embarrassment, and many indicated that they avoided sexual situations. Since most of these men had normal testosterone levels, and since they responded differently to sex questionnaires than normally potent men, Masters and Johnson concluded that impotence was primarily a psychological problem. What they missed was that the negative attitudes about sex stemmed from the impotence rather than causing it.

Sometimes a diagnosis of psychological impotence is clearcut, and no tests need to be done. The best example is the man who is unable to have sex with one partner, but is just fine with another. Another is the widower who has firm erections with masturbation, but is unable to achieve a good erection when he tries to have sex for the first time after his wife has passed away. This is actually quite a common story, with guilt and feelings of disloyalty playing a major role.

Another example is the fellow who informed me that every night he awakened with an excellent erection at around three A.M. and was able to have sex then with his girlfriend as long as she was willing. He insisted that for the last year he was unable to obtain a decent erection at any other time. His history was complicated in that he had been treated for prostate cancer with radiation, which can injure the nerves required for erection. He went through some tests, then announced at a follow-up visit that his erections were now fine during the daytime as well. If the penis can become properly erect at any one time, it means that the plumbing and wiring are okay, and that the source of the problem is between the ears. I tell patients that when it comes to sex, the mind is the only part of the body that can act like a faulty wire, sometimes on, sometimes off.

I see a great many men who have clearly adjusted well emotionally to their impotence. They may be successful at work, happy in their marriage, and may have discovered new ways to enjoy sex with their partners. However, the smile on their faces after successful treatment of impotence gives the lie to the assertion that a lack of erections does not affect them. I believe it affects men profoundly, and I have grown accustomed to hearing how men's attitudes in all spheres of their lives have improved once they are able to be sexual again in a manner that feels familiar and correct to them. For this reason, I encourage men to seek solutions to impotence. The benefits may extend beyond the bedroom.

■ NERVE DAMAGE

Men with diseases or injuries that affect the nerves may be prone to impotence. This includes men with multiple sclerosis and with spinal cord injuries. These men will often obtain completely rigid erections, but may be unable to control when they occur. These erections occur as a reflex to stimulation, but since they are often short-lived, they are not useful for intercourse. Erections can occur if the nerves in and around the penis are undamaged, but if the nerve connection to the brain is injured, there can be no connection between arousal and erection. Men with spinal cord injuries may also have no feeling in the genital region, which reduces the physical pleasure associated with sex.

The nerves controlling erections may be injured by a number of operations, such as those performed on the prostate, bladder, or rectum, since the nerves travel near these structures. Radiation to the pelvis may also damage nerves and result in impotence. In these cases the blood supply to the penis and the blood-trapping mechanism may work just fine. Indeed, some treatments with medications work so well in men with nerve damage that they require extra care to avoid erections that will not go away.

■ DIAGNOSIS AND EVALUATION OF IMPOTENCE

The first part of any medical evaluation is to establish the history of the problem and conduct a physical exam. If the impotence has been present for more than twelve months, if it has been progressive, or if it has occurred within a stable relationship, then the chances are great that there is a physical problem. If the problem has been more intermittent, with occasionally good and occasionally poor erections, then the likelihood is that the cause of the impotence is psychological.

When I do a physical exam for impotence, I focus primarily on the genital region, although I also look for breast enlargement or unusually sparse body hair, which may indicate a hormonal abnormality. I examine the penis for areas of internal scar tissue, and I check the testicles for size and firmness. I make sure the pulses in the groin are strong, and I do a rectal exam to feel the prostate and to assess the nerves in the area.

If the history suggests a physical basis for impotence, I will obtain blood tests. Testosterone levels are important for reasons discussed earlier. Blood count and chemistries are useful screening tests for a variety of medical disorders that may contribute to impotence. If the sugar is high in the blood, this might be a sign of diabetes, which is often a cause of impotence.

A useful test to help determine whether there is a physical basis to the erection problem is the sleep study described above. I almost always perform this test if it seems the problem is partly psychological, or if I think it will be useful to obtain information on the quality of nighttime erections.

In many cases I perform sophisticated blood-vessel studies. One test, called ultrasound, measures the flow of blood within the arteries of the penis. In the flaccid condition there is little flow in these arteries. However, by injecting medicine into the penis with a tiny needle, the penis can be "activated," and blood flow through the arteries increases dramatically. This mimics what happens during a normal erection. If the flow of blood after injection is low, it indicates an arterial blood-supply problem. A second test called cavernosometry shows how well the penis traps the blood entering the corpora cavernosa. Dye is then injected to see which channels the blood may be taking to escape. Neither of these tests is particularly uncomfortable, and they provide critical information to determine whether the problem is due to inflow, poor trapping, or both. Proper treatment obviously requires proper diagnosis.

■ TREATMENT OF IMPOTENCE—MEDICATIONS

Ideally, there would be a simple pill, or perhaps even better, a magical incantation, that would restore one's penis to the glory days of youth. Pills do exist, but there is no evidence that they do any real good. The best known and most widely used medication is called yohimbine, which is a natural derivative of a tree bark. Although I have had a small number of patients who say yohimbine has helped them, it has never been shown in any study to be effective for physical impotence. Since the side effects are minimal, my main objection to it is that it is a waste of time and money, especially since effective treatments are available.

Hope for an effective pill for impotence was spurred by the

publication of the following story in a medical journal. A psychiatrist in Montreal felt depressed and decided to treat himself with an antidepressant medication called trazodone. He also happened to be single and impotent, and whenever he took his trazodone, he could achieve a decent erection within the next several hours. Although he gave up using the medication for his depression, he began taking it with good success before going out on dates. He finally sought medical help for his depression and told his trazodone story. The psychiatrist was given sleep tests after taking either the trazodone or a placebo, but not knowing which. Only poor erections were seen with the placebo, but normal erections appeared with the trazodone. Naturally, this story created tremendous interest in an "impotence pill." However, further studies have demonstrated that it works in only a very small number of men. Nevertheless, it seems hopeful that other medications may be developed that will work more effectively.

Another false hope that failed in an amusing way was nitropaste. This is a cream containing nitroglycerin that is applied directly to the skin, used in the treatment of heart disease. Nitropaste causes blood vessels to swell, which is similar to the mechanism of a normal erection. It seemed natural, then, to try nitropaste for impotent men, applied directly to the penis. Although some men did achieve modest improvement in their erections, the trial failed in part because many of the women partners complained of headaches, a common side effect of nitropaste. The medication on the penis was rapidly absorbed by the women through the vagina. Suffice to say, there is as yet no effective pill or cream to improve erections, although this may change within the next ten years.

■ INJECTIONS

In 1982 it was discovered that injection of a medicine called papaverine into the penis caused an erection and could be used to treat impotence. This discovery changed the face of impotence, since there now existed an effective nonsurgical treatment. Over the last decade considerable experience has been gathered with papaverine as well as other medications for the treatment of impotence.

Whenever I mention penile injections to men who have never heard of it, they always look at me sideways as if I were joking. "You want me to do what?" they say. In fact, although the idea of putting a needle into the penis may seem bizarre and frightening, it is painless, takes only a few moments, and is very effective. It is relatively painless because the shaft of the penis is not particularly sensitive to pain. Of course, it is pleasantly sensitive to the light touch of sexual stimulation, but it takes a fair amount of pressure or pinching to elicit pain.

For an injection, a tiny needle is placed into the side of the penis (not the sensitive glans), and the medicine is expelled into the corpora cavernosa with the plunger. After the needle is withdrawn, pressure is held at the injection site for thirty seconds so that no bleeding or bruising results. After five to ten minutes the penis starts filling, and rigidity occurs several minutes later. The medication works by allowing the arteries supplying the corpora cavernosa to swell and provide increased blood flow, while at the same time it activates the trapping mechanism within the penis.

Although papaverine was the first agent used for this purpose and is still the most commonly used, I prefer a medication called prostaglandin E1 (PGE1). This medication appears to be more effective than papaverine alone and is safer. The side effects of papaverine include prolonged erections, abnormalities of liver enzymes, and internal scarring, which can result in worsening erections or curvature of the penis. These side effects are all much less common with PGE1.

Many men now use injections in order to have adequate erections for intercourse. It may take a few injections before they are comfortable with the technique, but it is not difficult at all. Once a proper dosage has been determined, patients complete a training session on how to inject themselves. Although the technique is effective for most impotent men, it is not universally successful. A combination of several medications may be necessary for men who do not achieve a firm enough erection with PGE1 alone.

The downside to injection therapy is the inconvenience of needing to draw up medication and to inject oneself every time one wants to have sex. In addition, PGE1 must be refrigerated to maintain its shelf life, so that traveling becomes more problematic. Apart from these considerations, injections provide an excellent nonsurgical option for impotent men.

■ THE PENILE PROSTHESIS

Some form of device or material has been used surgically to add stiffness to the penis since the early 1950s, but it took a while to find a reasonable way to do it. The first material used was cartilage, placed under the skin of the penis to mimic the baculum, a bone found in the penis of several mammals, including the walrus and the fox. The problem with cartilage was that without a blood supply of its own it was rapidly broken down by the body. Plastic splints placed beneath the penile skin provided rigidity fairly well, but were cosmetically unacceptable. Men with such a device walked around with what appeared to be a flagpole in their pants, since there was no mechanism to take the penis out of its "position of function."

The first real advance came with the development of cylindrical plastic implants, or prostheses, with metal cores that could bend, and these were placed inside each of the corpora cavernosa. These implants gave the penis stiffness so that penetration could be achieved and also allowed the penis to be bent for concealment under clothing.

The next advance in the early 1970s was an inflatable device consisting of a pump, reservoir, and two hollow cylinders. The cylinders were placed inside the corpora cavernosa, and the pump was placed within the scrotum like a small third testicle. When squeezed, the pump transferred fluid from a reservoir behind the pubic bone into the cylinders. A deflation valve allowed the transfer of fluid back out of the cylinders. Some men listen to descriptions of inflatable devices and say the process seems complicated. However, all that is required is to find the pump in the scrotum and give it a few squeezes. There are now sneakers that are more complicated than this.

Although they require more surgery, inflatable implants have become quite popular since they mimic the natural action of the penis. Modern inflatable devices are conceptually identical to the early models, although there have been technical improvements to minimize mechanical problems such as kinked tubing or leakage of fluid. The mechanical failure rate requiring reoperation is now very low, with overall patient satisfaction well over 90 percent.

There are still implants that do not inflate. These have also improved over the last several years and are a good option for many men. Since these are fairly pliable, concealment is not a significant issue. Despite this, they have enough rigidity to make penetration possible. The main advantage of the noninflatable prostheses is that little can go wrong. The main risk for all implants is infection, but this is uncommon.

The disadvantage of the noninflatable devices is that the penis may not get as full as with the inflatable devices, and that when undressed, the penis partly stands out. The inflatable devices give an excellent cosmetic appearance in both the inflated and deflated conditions. One widower with an inflatable implant proudly told me that his girlfriend was unaware that he had an implant at all.

Penile implants of the inflatable or noninflatable type must still be considered the gold-standard treatment for impotence. They have been around a long time and have an excellent track record. Several models are available, made by different manufacturers, and a device can be selected appropriate for the patient. Exactly what is involved?

Inserting a penile prosthesis can take from one to three hours,

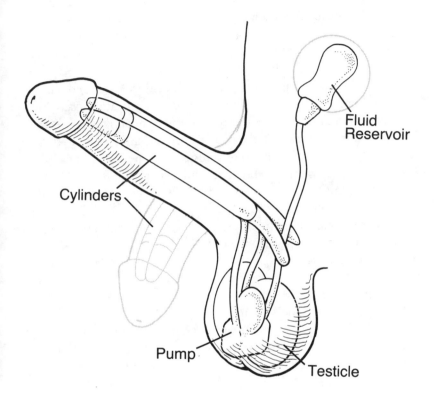

Fluid Reservoir

Cylinders

Pump

Testicle

The inflatable penile prosthesis consists of two cylinders within the penis, a fluid reservoir placed in the pelvis, and a pump in the scrotum. Squeezing the round portion of the pump transfers fluid from the reservoir into the penile cylinders, and a firm erection occurs. To deflate, a bar at the bottom of the pump is pressed, and fluid returns from the cylinders to the reservoir.

depending on the surgeon and the type of implant. I do the procedure under general or spinal anesthesia and keep my patients in the hospital overnight. There is moderate discomfort for about two weeks, particularly underneath the scrotum where the deep end of the penis lies. It takes four to six weeks before I give my patients the green light to have sex.

The main advantage of implants is that they work and work well. In general, my happiest impotence patients are those who have chosen an implant, since after the initial healing, sex is easy and requires no fuss. The downside of implants is that they require surgery, with a period of soreness and healing afterward. Although in general the erection obtained with an implant is very good, the penis will probably not be quite as long or as thick as it had been in one's youth.

Few men are unhappy afterward, but those that are almost always had expectations that were too high. Some men think that being able to have sex again is going to fix their relationships, make them instantly attractive to the opposite sex, or make their lives turn out better for some mystical reason. Obviously, having something firm in one's pants is not answer enough for life's trials. The bottom line is that the implant does one thing only, but does it well. It gives the penis enough rigidity to perform sexually. Expectations beyond this lead to disappointment.

■ VASCULAR SURGERY

Two types of blood-vessel problems may contribute to impotence: arterial disease may restrict inflow, or insufficient blood may be trapped due to venous leak. For men with venous leaks, the major veins draining the penis can be tied off. This operation, available for the last eight years or so, is called a venous ligation.

Success rates for venous ligation of the penis have been 50 percent at best. So far it has not been possible to identify beforehand those men who are most likely to benefit. Among those who benefit greatly from the procedure, a significant proportion will then fail over the next one to two years, either through worsening of the underlying venous leak or by the development of new channels for drainage of blood.

Another operation for men with a venous leak or with arterial disease is a bypass. In my experience, this seems to have a greater success rate than venous ligation, and it also makes more sense to me. Essentially, the goal is to provide more inflow by hooking up another artery to the penis. The artery I use is one of several that deliver blood to the lower abdominal muscles. At surgery this artery is connected to one of the blood vessels in the penis using the operating microscope. The result is analogous to having an additional fuel line hooked up to the engine. The veins are tied off as well, so that the patient benefits by having better inflow combined with diminished outflow.

This procedure is generally performed on younger men (under sixty), who seem to have a better chance of success. As men age, the likelihood of atherosclerosis in multiple blood vessels increases, which may diminish the results of the procedure. Since there is a larger incision, extending up the lower abdomen, there is more discomfort than for the venous ligation, and a stay in the hospital of two to three days is standard. Success rates in the range of 60 to 70 percent are to be expected, with even better results among men under forty with only an arterial injury.

Mike was a fifty-eight-year-old computer programmer who had been unable to achieve a decent erection for over five years. He and his wife engaged in mutual manual and oral sex, but Mike found this unsatisfactory. His arterial studies showed poor flow into the penis, and cavernosometry showed a large venous leak. He had both an inflow and a trapping problem. Mike was dead set against anything "artificial" in his body, such as an implant, and he did not care for injections. What to do? Mike opted to try the bypass operation.

A few weeks after surgery I saw Mike back in my office. I asked him how he was feeling, how his incisions had healed, and so on. He finally interrupted me. "Doc, don't you want to know the good stuff? I've had a solid erection every morning when I wake up, and I've had sex with my wife twice this week already." One year after his surgery, Mike continues to have decent erections and is very pleased he went through the operation. Vascular surgery such as the bypass is a good option for many men as long as they understand that the chances of success are good but far from perfect. The man looking for a "sure thing" would be better off with an implant.

■ VACUUM ERECTION DEVICES

An effective noninvasive way to achieve an erection is to use something called a vacuum erection device. A plastic cylinder is placed over the penis, and air is pumped out of the cylinder. This creates a partial vacuum in the cylinder, which makes the penis fill up with blood. A reasonable erection can be produced in this way, and then a special rubber band is slipped onto the base of the penis to trap the blood and maintain the erection. The vacuum device is then removed, and the man is left with a firm penis with a band encircling the base. One minor drawback is that the band prevents semen from coming out the tip of the penis during ejaculation. The semen may seep out later or be washed out with urination.

This device works reasonably well, although in my practice it is less well liked than injections. The paraphernalia is bulkier, a fair amount of lubrication must be used on the penis and against the pubic bone to create a good air seal, and the penis looks a little bluish with this method. The device costs approximately $400, although cheaper models are finding their way to market. For the man in a stable relationship who is averse to needles or surgery, vacuum devices may be a reasonable choice.

CHAPTER 6

PRIAPISM

■ Believe it or not, it is possible to have an erection that lasts too long. Curiously, these erections are not associated with sexual thoughts or sexual activity, and the penis does not soften after ejaculation. After four to six hours the penis becomes painful, which is when men are most likely to call their doctor or go to an emergency room. Although men are famous for bragging about real or imagined sexual prowess, few men brag about this problem to their buddies.

This condition is called priapism (pry-a-pism), named after the Greek god Priapus, who was the god of fertility and is depicted in pictures and statues with an enormous erect penis. Priapism occurs as a result of improper drainage of blood from the penis. As blood stagnates it becomes acidic, loses its oxygen, and the red blood cells then stiffen, making it even more difficult for them to squeeze out of the penis. If priapism is not treated in a timely fashion, scarring within the penis may eventually occur, and impotence is the final result. There are rare cases of gangrene of the penis resulting as well. Clearly, this is not a condition to be ignored.

Priapism does not occur because of excessive lovemaking or an unusually high level of sexual excitation. There is almost always a reason, whether it is a medical condition such as leukemia or some medication. Over the last ten years the most common cause of priapism has been the use of penile injections, usually in an inappropriate manner. Papaverine in particular can cause this problem. Some men foolishly increase the dose of medication without consulting their doctor, and priapism results. It is very unusual, however, for a man to develop priapism if he uses the dose prescribed by his physician. Apart from the obvious cases of self-injection of erection-producing agents, the most common offending agents are psychiatric medications, although the list of drugs reported to cause this condition is endless. It is unclear why some of these medications can produce priapism, although this is being studied to see if the lessons learned with priapism could be applied to improving erections in men with impotence.

Medical conditions that can make blood thicker or change the pliability of red blood cells can also cause priapism. Sickle-cell disease in boys is associated with priapism, presumably due to the change in shape of the red blood cells when they are exposed to lower concentrations of oxygen or an acid environment. These sickled cells jam up the pathways leading out of the penis, causing an erection that will not go away.

Priapism in boys or men with sickle-cell disease is generally treated by blood transfusions, to get normal blood into the penis and dilute the sick blood acting as a doorstop. In most other patients, the treatment is to place a needle in the side of the penis and drain out the dark, stagnant blood. Medication may be injected to shrink the blood vessels, reducing the inflow of blood. This takes care of the priapism in short order.

Before we knew as much about the control of erections, priapism was a complicated problem to treat, often requiring surgery to create pathways for blood to leave the penis. These procedures would eventually work, but there was a significant risk of impotence with such operations. It was also not nearly as effective, and the textbooks were full of creative ways to attack this problem.

I remember helping on such a case early in my training. The treatment took advantage of the fact that the glans, or head of the penis, is soft and unaffected in cases of priapism. The goal was therefore to make small connections between the corpora cavernosa and the glans so that blood could drain out. Following this particular operation the treatment appeared to be partially successful, in that the penis became less erect, but was still far from flaccid. It seemed that if left alone, the penis still had a tendency to fill and become erect, but if it were squeezed it would drain via the glans and become softer again. After surgery the patient was taken to an isolation room, and a nurse was instructed to inflate a blood pressure cuff placed around the penis every five minutes for the next eight hours. This worked, but I think it is fair to say this was a cumbersome treatment at best.

Though less than ten years old, the modern treatment of priapism has already rendered surgery essentially obsolete. The big difference was learning how erections worked so that a reasonable choice of medications could be used. The key is to use adrenaline or similar drugs that keep the penis flaccid by constricting the arterial inflow of blood. Once the answer is known, it always seems so simple!

CHAPTER 7

THE BENT PENIS

■ One of the most disturbing problems that can happen to a man is developing a bent penis. The curve can be so severe that intercourse may be impossible. This is most commonly due to a condition called Peyronie's disease. In Peyronie's disease internal scarring or fibrosis of the penis occurs, resulting in nodules beneath the skin, penile curvature with erections, or impotence.

The worst case of Peyronie's disease I ever heard of comes from a history book of urology, which reports how a nobleman took a swim in a river in winter, against the advice of his entourage. He developed such a cramp that his penis permanently curled up like a corkscrew. He held a stone tablet at his navel whenever he urinated, or else he would spray his face with urine. Although this example underscores the potential extent of curvature, I suspect that the eighteenth-century authors of this report may have taken certain liberties in their description, since Peyronie's disease has little effect on the flaccid penis. It is during erection that the curve becomes noticeable.

To explain what happens it is helpful to use again the analogy of a long balloon. If one places a piece of tape along part of the balloon and then inflates it, the balloon will curve around the piece of tape, since that area will not expand as much as the rest of the balloon. The same holds true in the penis affected by Peyronie's disease. The outer sheath of the corpora cavernosa becomes thickened and is unable to stretch due to scarring. As the penis expands, it curves around the area of the scar. Most commonly the scar tissue is on the top surface, and so the most common direction of curvature is up toward the navel. Several scarred areas may exist, however, and I have had patients whose erect penises were twisted like a corkscrew.

Men may go to see a doctor for one of several reasons if they have Peyronie's disease. The first is they may feel a lump within the penis and be worried about cancer. Cancer of the penis, however, always involves the skin and is quite unusual. If a deep lump is felt within the penis without any overlying skin abnormalities, this is likely to be Peyronie's disease. Another reason men come to the doctor with Peyronie's disease is that they are experiencing painful erections. There may not be any noticeable curvature yet, but the scarring limits the full expansion of the penis with erection, and this can be painful. The characteristic knot of tissue within the penis can usually be felt, although it may take weeks to months before it eventually shows up.

The most common complaint, though, is a penis that is bent with erections. The curvature may come on quite suddenly, with some men insisting that their penis was straight one night and bent the next. Some men will notice a narrowed area along the shaft rather than curvature, and others will complain of a penis that is firm at the base and soft at the tip. All of these may be due to Peyronie's, and all may coexist.

The cause of Peyronie's disease is unknown in most cases. In some men it is clearly the result of injury. Scott provides a good example. Scott described how his penis had buckled during intercourse with his girlfriend. He was sore at the time, but was able to continue having sex. A week later he awakened with a painful penis bending upward toward his navel at almost a right angle. The association of buckling injury and Peyronie's disease has made investigators wonder whether all cases are due to injury, perhaps occurring during sleep. Since men normally have multiple erections each night, perhaps a minor injury might occur by their turning over in their sleep onto a firm penis.

The response of the body to injury includes scarring, which produces tissue that will not stretch. If scarring of the inner penis occurs, blood will fail to be trapped properly, a venous leak occurs, and impotence may result. Occasionally, the fibrosis may extend all the way through one or both corpora cavernosa, blocking arterial inflow beyond the scar tissue, while at other times the scarring may also appear as a constriction of the penis, as if there were an invisible napkin ring around it. Most commonly, there is an oval of scar tissue that runs along the top surface of the penis, causing the erection to swing around it. Painful erections are an early and temporary part of the process. The pain resolves with time, probably due to the reduced pressures within the corpora cavernosa from a venous leak.

The treatment for most men is nothing more than reassurance that no terrible problem has befallen them. If a man is able to achieve firm erections adequate for intercourse, and the curvature does not interfere with lovemaking, then there is no need to do anything. If pain is the problem, knowing that this will go away over several months is often treatment enough.

Some men may benefit from taking vitamin E at a dose of six hundred to a thousand units daily. It is hard to say how well it works, since the curvature and pain of Peyronie's disease may resolve spontaneously. Nevertheless, some evidence suggests improvement for some men with vitamin E. The theoretical basis for using vitamin E is that it has a beneficial effect on the scarring process. Once the scarring has stabilized, however, no medicine will affect it. Another medicine called para-aminobenzoate has been used, but it is no more effective than vitamin E, and more unpleasant to take.

Surgery is reserved for severe cases where the curve interferes with intercourse, the quality of erections is poor, or rarely, when the nodules themselves cause an emotional problem for the patient. If erections are still good, it is reasonable to remove the plaque itself. The plaque includes the wall of the sheath covering the corpora cavernosa, so plaque removal also requires coverage of the cylinders with a graft. Some surgeons use skin taken from the hip or elsewhere on the body. I have preferred to use a synthetic material that has a little "give" to it, but is strong and readily available in the operating room, without the need for another wound.

When erections are of poor quality, it is unlikely that mere straightening of the penis will improve the ability to achieve adequate rigidity. In a small number of cases I have removed the plaque and also performed a venous ligation, with good success. For the most part, men with poor rigidity will do better with simultaneous placement of a penile prosthesis. These can be either inflatable or noninflatable, but either way these men will then have a straight, functional penis, which is the real goal of treatment.

CHAPTER 8

PREMATURE EJACULATION

■ Although not truly a medical condition, premature ejaculation causes considerable emotional distress for men and their partners. Strictly speaking, premature ejaculation refers to ejaculation taking place prior to actual placement of the penis within the vagina. More commonly, men complain of ejaculating quickly after penetration, and I think of this as premature ejaculation as well. The point is that little or no time is spent by the couple while they are genitally "engaged." Men may feel inadequate as lovers and may be concerned that their partners are angry or disappointed with them.

In essence, this is a social problem. The requirements of reproductive biology are satisfied once sperm are deposited within the vagina. Indeed, it is interesting to ponder why there should be any premium placed on prolonged sexual intercourse, as there clearly is in this culture. For the man, orgasm is a distinctly pleasurable event whether it follows a brief or extended period of sexual stimulation. For the woman, the major drawback to abbreviated intercourse is that there may be insufficient time to achieve orgasm. In terms of reproduction, however, does it matter whether women achieve orgasm? Many women who never experience orgasm become pregnant without difficulty. So, for reproductive purposes there is no absolute female requirement for orgasm as there is for men.

Nevertheless, orgasm is clearly a pleasurable experience for women, and achieving a climax may be an important part of a sexual encounter. This is not obvious to all men. Nor is it necessarily understood that sexual satisfaction for a woman can be achieved by clitoral stimulation without any genital contact at all. Failing to appreciate this can lead to frustration, disappointment, and tension within a sexual relationship.

Premature ejaculation is extremely common early in a man's sexual career. In most cases it resolves with time, experience, and with increased confidence in one's sexual abilities. For better or worse, as a man ages, his penis becomes less sensitive, and this tends to prolong the period of stimulation needed to produce an orgasm.

A variety of solutions have been offered for premature ejaculation, but most of them make little sense. A common one is to think about dying in order to stave off the dreaded early ejaculation. Interesting variants on this theme are to pinch oneself hard enough to cause pain, bite the inside of a cheek, or think about one's job or schoolwork. In other words, make sex unpleasant in order for it to last longer. Other solutions to desensitize the penis by anesthetic sprays or by wearing one or more condoms do not make much sense to me either. Since one of the major attractions of sex is that it is pleasurable, why make it less pleasurable?

A forty-one-year-old Greek restaurant owner, Nick, came to see me. He had been married for eighteen years and had three teenage children. One night after having sex with him, his wife burst into tears. When he asked her what was wrong, she told him that during their entire marriage she had never experienced an orgasm with him. She complained that he ejaculated too quickly, before she was satisfied. This sweet man was struck to his core. He clearly loved his wife very much, but had not paid much attention to her in sexual terms for many years. Not only had he disappointed his wife but his manhood was now in question as well. He admitted that throughout their marriage he had always climaxed within a few moments of penetration.

Nick had seen another urologist, who thought he would benefit from using penile injections. Although this did result in good rigidity even following ejaculation, Nick did not feel that this was a good option for him. His wife objected to his using needles and medicines for her benefit. What could I offer him?

The problem here is really one of timing. If his wife had not complained, Nick would have been happy to continue with a short period of sex leading to ejaculation. Nick now wanted to prolong intercourse only so that his wife could climax as well. Options to solve this problem included more foreplay directed at bringing Nick's wife closer to climax before penetration, or continuing to stimulate her following ejaculation. Nick indicated that due to their cultural and religious background, he could not manually stimulate his wife. Few choices were available. It was time for Nick to retrain his penis.

Ejaculation is complex and involves physical reflexes combined with emotional and psychological factors. Some men with premature or early ejaculation will not need to ejaculate despite prolonged pleasurable manual or oral stimulation, but will then climax within microseconds of having their penis within a vagina. These men underscore the point that there is more to ejaculation than merely receiving enough stimulation. For any man, the amount of stimulation needed to reach orgasm varies according to circumstances. Many men report that ejaculation occurs much sooner if they are particularly excited, or if there has been a long period between sex. The psychological aspect to sex and orgasm must be appreciated in treating premature ejaculation.

For most of Nick's life, his body and mind were accustomed to reach ejaculation immediately following vaginal penetration. And until recently, Nick never had any reason to try to change this pattern. Now he had some work to do.

I use a technique described by Masters and Johnson. The goal is twofold; one is to break the established pattern of penetration followed immediately by ejaculation, and the other is to gain mastery over the ejaculatory process. At some point during male sexual stimulation, ejaculation is about to happen and nothing can stop it. This is called the point of inevitability. With practice, a man can learn to sense when he is approaching the point of inevitability and can then do one of several things. He can reach that point and then ejaculate. If he is experienced in paying attention to his body, he can change gears and let the feeling slide away. Or he can use what is called the choke technique.

With the choke technique the shaft of the penis is grasped tightly just before the threshold for ejaculation is reached. Firm pressure will inhibit ejaculation, and sexual stimulation can be resumed when the feeling of impending ejaculation recedes. By repeating this technique, a man may postpone his ejaculation for some time. With practice, the time to reach the point of inevitability becomes delayed. More importantly, a sense of control over ejaculation emerges, bringing with it the confidence necessary to become more adept at mutual lovemaking.

I explained all of this to Nick. He grasped my hand and shook it several times before leaving the office that first day. "Doctor, you have given me hope again. I thought my marriage was lost. Thank you." I saw him again after he had practiced with his wife for a month. It was not working. Twice he had ejaculated before he could squeeze the penis. Another time he had successfully terminated the urge to ejaculate, but he had become flaccid and did not resume intercourse. I assured Nick this was all part of the usual trial and error. Two months later Nick walked in with some pastries. "Thank you for saving my marriage, Doctor. Everything works as you said it would."

For many men in stable relationships, the problem of timing can be addressed in more creative ways. Extended foreplay with increased attention directed toward one's partner can be a pleasurable solution to the partner's frustration with quick ejaculation. Many men are able to achieve a second erection after ejaculation with which they are less apt to ejaculate quickly. This may provide an adequate period of sex for mutual satisfaction. Finally, stimulation of one's partner can be continued after ejaculation if both parties are so inclined.

CHAPTER 9

PROSTATE PROBLEMS

■ A Slow Stream

As men reach their fifties, they often begin to notice that they no longer urinate with the force they once had. As men reach sixty, it becomes commonplace to urinate more frequently, and awakening at night to urinate becomes routine. This is usually due to benign growth of the prostate, called BPH for the technical term *benign prostatic hypertrophy*. Since the prostate sits at the opening of the bladder like a gatekeeper, it can significantly affect how forcefully and efficiently the bladder empties. As the prostate grows from the size of a chestnut to as large as an orange, it can compress the urethra passing through its center, making it more difficult for the urine to be squeezed out. The bladder muscle forces urine through the prostate, but much energy is expended to simply open up the sides of the enlarged prostate, which want to lie against each other. This reduces the force of the stream. The stream may come out as a dribble, in spurts, or it might even be necessary to push the urine out by straining the abdominal muscles.

As the prostate grows, it becomes increasingly difficult to push the prostate open and empty the bladder completely. A residual amount of urine remains, and a man may therefore sense that his bladder is never empty. He may need to return to the bathroom to urinate within minutes of doing so a first time and still void a substantial amount of urine the second time. If the bladder is never empty, it also takes less time to become full. Urinary frequency may then become a nuisance.

In some men the bladder responds to the enlarged prostate by becoming irritated, and there may be a tremendous urge to urinate all of a sudden. This urgency, especially when combined with the need to urinate frequently, can be annoying. Men may find they cannot stay on the job for more than an hour or two, or they must interrupt business meetings to get to the bathroom. Some men who do a lot of driving carry a jug in the car for frequent pit stops when the urge strikes them.

Worse situations may occur, however. Eventually, some men may be unable to void at all, a condition called urinary retention. The bladder fills and fills, but no more than a few drops come out. This causes considerable discomfort, and a trip to the emergency room may be necessary to drain the bladder by passing a tube through the urethra. This generally occurs only after a long period of progressively worsening urination. Some medications may precipitate retention, especially those designed to treat flu symptoms. These should be avoided if you have an enlarged prostate and a slow or frequent stream. It may also be difficult to urinate after surgery, but this problem almost always resolves if the prostate is not too large.

Another serious problem that may result from BPH is the development of stones in the bladder. These are completely different from stones in the gallbladder and have a different location and symptoms from kidney stones. When urine pools, as it does in a bladder that empties incompletely, the chemicals in the urine can form stones. These stones may cause bleeding or predispose to bladder infections. They can also interfere with urinating by intermittently blocking the opening of the bladder

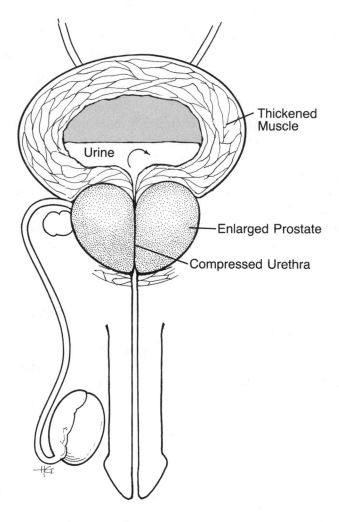

Thickened
Muscle

Urine

Enlarged Prostate

Compressed Urethra

When the prostate is enlarged, it compresses the urethra, making it more difficult for the bladder to squeeze out urine. The bladder muscle may become thickened. The force of urination is diminished, and there may be leftover urine in the bladder following urination. Frequent, slow urination is the usual result of an enlarged prostate.

like a ball valve. In the middle of urinating there might be a sudden stop to the stream, often accompanied by considerable discomfort.

Finally, some men may feel that they void reasonably well, but are actually walking around with a bladder always filled to at least 90 percent. The pressure in the bladder may be elevated, causing backpressure on the kidneys. The kidneys swell, and their function may deteriorate.

Generally speaking, men with symptoms of urinary retention, bladder stones, recurrent infections, and BPH causing kidney trouble should all have surgery performed to allow the urine to empty freely from the bladder. This is done by removing the inner part of the prostate, so that the urethra is no longer compressed between the lobes of the prostate. However, most men who undergo prostate surgery for BPH do not have any of these more serious conditions. For the most part, surgery is performed for the nuisance symptoms described above, in order to improve the quality of their lives.

This is an important point, since quality-of-life issues are different for everyone. I have seen men in the office who were miserable because they had to wake up twice a night to urinate and felt that it interfered with their activities the following day. I have had other patients who awakened every hour but who felt that this was not a serious problem for them. The first patient should consider surgery, and the second patient should not. The size of the prostate is not important in deciding whether or not to operate. It really comes down to symptoms, and how much they affect the quality of a man's life.

Surgery is effective in improving the force of the stream, reducing the time it takes to void, and even reducing the amount of dribbling that occurs after voiding. It also tends to reduce the number of times men wake up at night, but this is not always so. The reason is that the bladder undergoes some changes from working against a blockage for so many years. The muscle of the bladder responds to the blockage by becoming thicker, just as arm muscles become thicker after regular workouts. The thickened bladder is prone to urinating more frequently than a normal bladder, even after the blockage has been removed.

Two types of operations are most commonly performed for enlarged prostates. Both are designed to remove the central part of the prostate and leave the outer portion alone. I think of this as removing the meat from an orange and leaving the peel behind. Before the advent of today's telescopes with excellent lenses and fiber-optic light sources, prostate surgery was performed most commonly through an incision in the lower abdomen. Today, this procedure is reserved for men with enormous prostates.

Over 90 percent of prostate surgery for BPH is now done through a telescope passed through the urethra. This is called a TURP, standing for *t*rans*u*rethral *r*esection of the *p*rostate. General or spinal anesthesia is used so there is no discomfort during the procedure. The surgeon looks inside the prostate and the bladder, and then carves out the inner portions of the prostate using an electrocautery device. At the end of the procedure a catheter, or soft plastic tube, allows the bloody urine to drain into a bag. Once the urine is clear, the catheter is removed and the patient goes home.

The TURP is a common, straightforward procedure, although it takes considerable skill to be performed properly by the urologist. The technical difficulty lies in being able to operate in a three-dimensional space through the two-dimensional view afforded by a telescope. The procedure takes roughly one to one and a half hours. There is remarkably little discomfort postoperatively. This is partly due to the fact that no skin incision has been made. The only wound is the raw inner surface of the prostate, which has little sensation.

The operation to remove the prostate with an abdominal incision, called an open prostatectomy, is now reserved for men with enormous prostates. Since the prostate is removed piecemeal during a TURP, the larger the prostate, the longer it takes to complete the procedure. With very large prostates the risk of bleeding is increased as well. Open prostatectomies take roughly the same amount of time regardless of the size of the prostate, usually around two hours. The downside is a longer stay in the hospital, up to a week, with more postoperative discomfort than after a TURP, since the incision must heal as well.

Although prostate surgery is frequently performed and usually goes smoothly, certain risks are associated with it. These include injury to the sphincter muscle next to the prostate, so that uncontrollable leakage of urine may occur. This is quite uncommon, unless there has been previous nerve damage, such as from a stroke. There is also a small risk of impotence from injury to nearby nerves. Scar tissue at the opening of the bladder or farther along the urethra may restrict the flow of urine and may need to be stretched open afterward.

Most men after prostate surgery will have retrograde ejaculation, in which the sperm and fluid pass back into the bladder rather than out the tip of the penis. This happens because the opening to the bladder is made so large that the fluid takes the path of least resistance, which is backward. This causes no physical problems, and the sensation of orgasm is unchanged. Making babies is more complicated as a result, but men who undergo this procedure are generally older and are no longer thinking about adding to their families.

■ ALTERNATIVE TREATMENTS FOR ENLARGED PROSTATES

A great number of men undergo TURP in the United States each year. It is the second-largest surgical expenditure in the Medicare budget. Once a man reaches age fifty, the chances are 20 percent that he will eventually undergo a prostate operation. These huge numbers have spurred interest in alternative means to treat BPH. Some of these are reasonable, and others are entirely experimental and may not pan out despite promising early results.

Medications

Currently two types of medication are available in the United States that are helpful to some men with symptoms of BPH. The first relaxes the smooth muscle around the prostate and bladder opening, and is prescribed as prazosin (Minipres) or terazosin (Hytrin). Modest improvement in voiding symptoms occurs in a third of patients. Since it does not shrink the prostate, the medication must be taken forever, or until prostate surgery is performed. It is reasonable to try this medication to avoid or delay surgery. Often it is clear that surgery is the best option, and in those instances I do not encourage taking these medications.

Shrinking the prostate is possible, but until recently this has not been an attractive option. Removing the hormone testosterone from the system will shrink the prostate about 30 percent, and this may improve symptoms considerably in some men. The most effective way to do this is by removal of the testicles, and in fact this was done around the turn of the century for men unable to urinate at all because of their enlarged prostates. This would not be a popular treatment now.

Medical ways to block the production or effects of testosterone are now available, with similar results but fewer side effects. A new medication called finasteride (Proscar) is now available. Testosterone levels and sexual performance remain unchanged, but the byproduct that stimulates prostate growth is blocked by the medication, and the prostate shrinks. Early results indicate that approximately one-third of men with enlarged prostates have improvement with this medication, generally men with only mild to moderate symptoms. Finasteride may prove to be a very useful medication, and urologists are quickly gaining experience with it. The full benefit of the medication may require up to six months of treatment. One concern is that it lowers the blood levels of PSA, which is used to detect prostate cancer, making interpretation of this test more difficult.

Surgical Procedures

A new procedure using a balloon to stretch open the prostate became quite popular for several years, but much of the early enthusiasm is now waning. The procedure was developed by a radiologist in Vancouver, Canada, who had significant voiding symptoms, but was reluctant to undergo surgery. He had experience with a technique to treat blockages in arteries with a long, thin balloon. He had the idea of treating his prostate the same way, but he could not find a urologist willing to try it. So he did it himself.

He passed a wire into his bladder through the urethra, then passed the special balloon over the wire, monitoring its position by X ray. When the balloon was within the prostate, he inflated it for several minutes. After several days his stream was somewhat improved. He repeated the procedure on himself with greater expansion of the balloon and found that his stream improved even more. His experience stimulated considerable interest, and special balloons have now been developed for this purpose. Despite the good result achieved by the radiologist on himself, there have been only mixed results for larger groups of patients. There is little evidence to suggest that balloon dilation of the prostate is an improvement over established treatments for enlarged prostates.

Newer procedures gearing up across the country are treatment of the prostate with laser and also with microwave radiation. The idea is to heat up the inner portion of the prostate enough so that the tissue becomes "cooked" and falls away, leaving a larger channel for the urine to pass through the prostate. Both these techniques are experimental and available only in a small number of centers around the country. Time will tell if they are reasonable alternatives to current therapy. In the meantime, it is good to remember that excellent treatment for BPH already exists.

Some men who develop urinary retention are too ill to undergo the risks of a surgical procedure. They may have severe heart or lung disease or may be dying of cancer. In the past, these men have had no choice but to have a catheter for the remainder of their lives. Over the last two years I have used an experimental technique to allow many of these men to urinate naturally without the need for a catheter. A small metal spring, called a prostate stent, is placed in the prostate to keep the passageway open. The stent eventually becomes covered with the normal internal lining and is incorporated into the body. The stent is placed through a telescope under local anesthesia. Results in more than twenty patients have been excellent, with nearly all men able to urinate freely. Although the prostate stent does not seem to improve urination to the same extent as a TURP, it does offer hope for a catheter-free existence for men too frail to undergo formal surgery.

■ PROSTATE CANCER

There has been a great deal of interest lately in prostate cancer. In fact, prostate cancer has been a hot topic over the last decade. It is a curious disease. On the one hand, more men die of prostate cancer than any other cancer except lung cancer. On the other hand, the vast majority of prostate cancers never cause any symptoms and are not responsible for deaths. The explanation for this paradox is that the disease is extremely common in older men and tends to grow very slowly. So, many men may have prostate cancer without knowing it and may die from other illnesses before the prostate cancer catches up to them. However, in some men prostate cancer grows more rapidly and can then cause trouble. For men in their fifties and sixties it may be particularly important to diagnose prostate cancer, since it would be worthwhile to treat even if it takes twenty years to become symptomatic.

Prostate cancer tends to grow so very slowly that even men with metastatic disease, when the cancer has spread to the bones or lungs, may live a trouble-free life for many years. On the other hand, aggressive cancers of the prostate do exist and may prove fatal within a year or less. Clearly, it is critical to diagnose prostate cancer in men in their fifties and sixties. In my opinion, it is also advisable to diagnose and treat men who are in good condition in their seventies. It may be less important to make the diagnosis for men in their eighties. I say this because as men reach their advanced years, the likelihood is high that they will die of other problems before a prostate cancer has the chance to do any harm.

The diagnosis of prostate cancer is most commonly made by physical examination. The rectal exam is an important part of the physical exam for this reason, particularly among men over fifty. No one likes it, but it is a mistake not to have it done. On several occasions I have detected prostate cancers in prominent individuals referred for other reasons, and where the referring physician had been reluctant to perform a rectal exam so as not to embarrass the patient. Shortcuts, even well-intentioned ones, can lead to tragedies.

The normal prostate is felt through the lining of the rectum as a firm, fleshy mass. A hard area may indicate cancer. Subtle signs of early prostate cancer may be a slightly firmer area, or one side of the prostate may be larger than the other. The rectal exam, the best test for prostate cancer, should be performed yearly on every man over fifty.

A recent addition to the physician's armamentarium in detecting prostate cancer is a blood test called prostate specific antigen, or PSA. This chemical is made only by the prostate, so diseases of other organs should not affect it. When the PSA is elevated, it generally indicates one of two things. Either the prostate is significantly enlarged, or prostate cancer is present. Infections of the prostate may also raise PSA levels temporarily.

Faced with a diagnosis of a possible prostate cancer, many men will respond by saying that it seems unlikely to them since they have no symptoms. One of the hallmarks of early prostate cancer is that there are no symptoms. Once symptoms appear, it is all too often at an advanced stage where cure is no longer possible. Advanced prostate cancer may cause bone pain, blockage of the kidneys, or blockage of the bladder opening just like BPH. Another blood test called acid phosphatase is frequently elevated when there has been spread of prostate cancer. In late stages there may be weakness or weight loss, as occurs with any advanced disease. The goal, of course, is to find cancers at an early stage while they are still curable.

Once there is a suspicion of a prostate cancer, either by elevated PSA or by physical examination, the next step is a biopsy. The biopsy is now most commonly performed together with an ultrasound of the prostate. The ultrasound uses a probe placed in the rectum and provides a clear picture of the prostate and nearby structures. Suspicious areas are noted, and then a small needle takes a sliver of prostate from these areas. The biopsy is felt as a small pinch. Several biopsies are the rule. The entire exam and biopsy last no more than fifteen to twenty minutes, after which most normal activities can be resumed.

The slivers of prostate tissue removed by the biopsy needle are examined under the microscope by a pathologist. If no cancer is seen, then follow-up is limited to yearly examinations and PSA tests. If cancer is diagnosed, then it is necessary to find out whether there is evidence of spread. A bone scan and chest X ray are routine, and other X rays may be performed as well.

For a healthy man with no evidence of cancer beyond his prostate, the best treatment is surgery to remove the entire prostate together with the cancer. Cure rates for localized disease are excellent. Radiation has also been used to treat prostate cancer, but the long-term results are not as good as surgery. Since radiation is less stressful than surgery in the short term, I do recommend it for men with significant health problems, and for most men older than seventy-five. Once the cancer has spread, there is no cure, although some treatments may slow down the disease. However, surgery to remove the prostate makes no sense if cancer cells are already in other parts of the body.

Surgery for prostate cancer is called radical prostatectomy and differs from surgery for benign enlargement of the prostate in several ways. The most important is that the entire prostate must be removed, which can only be done through an incision. This is considerably more complicated, since it means also removing the segment of the urethra that courses through the center of the prostate. A new connection between bladder and the remaining urethra must be made. The lymph nodes in the pelvis are also removed, since this is a common place for prostate cancer to spread.

Until the early 1980s urologists shied away from this operation due to two common complications. One is that a significant number of men were incontinent afterward, meaning that they had little or no control over urination. The sphincter muscle that keeps men dry is adjacent to the prostate, and if it is injured, urine will leak out constantly. The second complication was that nearly all men became completely impotent. The reason for this is that the nerves controlling erection lie just next to the prostate on either side, and they would be cut during surgery.

The major surgical advance for prostate cancer of the last ten years was the development of a technique whereby the sphincter muscle and the nerves could be clearly identified and preserved. Permanent incontinence is now quite unusual, although everyone has some leakage for as long as several months. A majority of men under age sixty-five have return of normal sexual function if the nerves were preserved as well.

Men with advanced prostate cancer are treated by lowering the levels of testosterone in the body. This is because most prostate cancer cells require testosterone to grow. By removing testosterone from the body, the cancer shrinks. The simplest way to lower testosterone levels is to remove the hormone-producing part of the testicles by a small outpatient procedure. Medical ways to produce the same effect include injections of medicine on a monthly basis. Even with spread of the disease, however, men may live for many years without missing a beat. One of the best examples is a patient of mine named Sam.

Sam first came to see me four years ago about poor erections. He was seventy-eight years old, his wife had died two years earlier, and he now had a girlfriend with whom he wanted to have intercourse. When I examined Sam, he appeared to be in excellent condition, but I noticed a hard lump on his prostate. When I mentioned this to him, he told me that a urologist had done some tests on his prostate three years earlier, and a decision was made to do nothing about it.

Upon obtaining Sam's old records I learned that a biopsy of the prostate had revealed cancer, and tests indicated the disease had already spread beyond the prostate. Yet Sam felt perfectly fine. He was also very clear that he wanted a penile prosthesis for treatment of his impotence. I repeated all of his blood tests and X rays. There was no evidence of further spread of the cancer. Sam had his surgery for a penile prosthesis and has been grateful to me ever since. I see him twice a year, and he has not had a single problem from his prostate apart from some slowing of his stream. He has sex with his girlfriend about twice a month, continues to work as a clerk, and seems quite pleased with his life.

The good news about prostate cancer is that it is a curable disease if diagnosed early, and our ability to detect it is improving. Even when the cancer has spread, there is often a long period without symptoms. I suspect that over the next decade there will be improved treatments for prostate cancer that has spread to other parts of the body.

CONCLUSION

■ The human body is amazing in its intricacies and design. Nowhere is this more true than with the male genitalia. Sperm production and delivery, erections, and urination are marvelous examples of engineering, benefiting from eons of evolution. However, together with the beautiful complexity of normal functioning goes the possibility of a breakdown in the system. This may result in a medical illness or impotence or infertility.

I have attempted in these pages to explain the normal anatomy and function of the male genital system, and also to describe many of the physical problems that can occur. My principal objective has been to educate, since knowledge is the main weapon we have against the fears and prejudices fostered by ignorance. An improved understanding of how your body works may be all you need to keep a minor problem in perspective. On the other hand, I have also tried to stress what types of problems or symptoms merit medical attention.

I hope that many of you who read this book will have a better understanding about a particular problem you might have. The fields of male infertility, impotence, and diseases of the prostate are moving ahead rapidly, and older texts are now outdated. If you have a question or problem that is not adequately covered in this book, I strongly urge you to speak to your doctor. You should regard your doctor not only as someone to see when you are ill but also as a resource for information. In my opinion, the best physicians are those who enjoy teaching about health, as well as caring for their patients when they are ill.

ACKNOWLEDGMENTS

■ This book was conceived roughly at the same time as my daughter Maya, and has grown in fits and starts between the obligations of clinical practice, academic papers, and running out to the store for an emergency supply of diapers. Somehow, my wife, Sue, managed to keep us all moving forward with her energy, love, and encouragement. Her superb editing helped keep me on track whenever I was inclined to wade into the dense jargon of medical terminology. Without her help, this project would never have matured into any semblance of a finished manuscript. The joy of seeing Maya born and watching her grow has made me appreciate in the most intimate way the wonders of reproduction and development.

It is an unusual family that consists entirely of accomplished writers. Throughout the many stages of my work, I benefited greatly from the advice, experience, and enthusiasm of my mother, Chawa Rosenfarb, my father, Dr. Henry Morgentaler, and my sister, Goldie Morgentaler. Their support was invaluable to me, especially at those times when the idea of finishing the book seemed an insurmountable task.

I wish to thank my editor, Gail Winston, for first proposing this project to me. She understood the need for an accessible book about men's health, and helped bring it about with her insightful editorial comments and suggestions. Finally, I must thank my mentor and colleague, William C. DeWolf, M.D., for his unwavering support in all my professional endeavors.

INDEX

ABOUT THE AUTHOR

■ Abraham Morgentaler, M.D., was born in Montreal, Canada, in 1956. He moved to Cambridge, Massachusetts, in 1974 to attend Harvard College, where he graduated magna cum laude. There he developed his interest in biology, studying the effects of hormones on the sexual behavior of lizards. He graduated from Harvard Medical School in 1982 and joined the staff at the Beth Israel Hospital in Boston, where he is the director of the Male Infertility and Impotency Program. Dr. Morgentaler is assistant professor of surgery (urology) at Harvard Medical School. He is an active researcher in the fields of male reproduction and sexual behavior. He currently lives with his family in the Boston area.